Of
This
Much
I'm
Sure

Of
This
Much
I'm
Sure

A memoir by

NADINE KENNEY JOHNSTONE

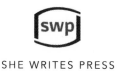

SHE WRITES PRESS

Published 2017
Printed in the United States of America
Print ISBN: 978-1-63152-210-9
E-ISBN: 978-1-63152-211-6
Library of Congress Control Number: 2016954306

For information, address:
She Writes Press
1563 Solano Ave #546
Berkeley, CA 94707

Cover design © Julie Metz, Ltd./metzdesign.com
Book design by Stacey Aaronson

She Writes Press is a division of SparkPoint Studio, LLC.

Names and identifying characteristics have been changed to protect the privacy of certain individuals.

For my boys.

Prologue

I never imagined that IVF might kill me.

But as the doctors rush me into emergency surgery, and Jamie whispers *I love you* like he fears he will never hold me again, a third of my blood volume pumps not through my veins but into my body, poisoning my organs.

I understand that these breaths might be my last.

Just before the anesthesia kicks in, what grips me is the irony—that this quest we've embarked on to create life might be the very thing that ends my own.

I will die young. I will die childless. I will die just when I've pushed everyone away.

And if I do live to survive, I am acutely aware that my life will forever be categorized as *before IVF* and *after.*

Here is the part of the story that Jamie and I always omit from the telling of our traumatic tale. After the egg retrieval, we didn't go straight to our house for me to rest, as directed. Almost twenty eggs had just been extracted from my ovaries and were being inseminated in a petri dish while I recovered. A pair of those fertilized embryos would be inserted into my uterus in three days, and I would be what I had wanted to be for so long: pregnant.

But then we made a stop on the way home from the clinic after the egg retrieval, and I will forever wonder if this pause in our journey changed our fate. It makes me question if I am to blame for the terror I faced that October Tuesday and the weeks, months, years that followed.

What detour could have been so important that it caused us to ignore doctors' orders? The pharmacy? The grocery store? No and no. The destination was Orchard House—Louisa May Alcott's home in Concord, Massachusetts, where she wrote her autobiographical novel, *Little Women*.

Every Christmas, I used to watch the movie version of the book and pine after the sort of life the March family had in the 1800s. I, too, wanted the warmth of a fireplace, the creak of old wood floors, furniture strewn with handmade quilts, hot cider for sipping. I craved cinnamon Bundt cakes and orange-glazed roasts. I ached to sing carols to the chords of my sister's piano playing.

Instead, we spent the Christmas Eves of my youth in our cold basement that Mom made festive with dollar-store stockings and plastic candy canes. Our windows fogged, not from the heat of a hearth, but from clouds of cigarette smoke. Dinner was South Side Chicago grub—Italian beef sandwiches, fried chicken, mostaccioli. In lieu of carols and piano tunes, my drunk uncles clanked bottles of Jager and called each other "jag-offs." My prepubescent cousins and I played dress-up, but rather than donning bonnets and lace gowns like the March girls, we stuffed socks into our plaid dresses and smeared our mouths with lipstick. To entertain the family, we belted out made-up songs with lyrics like: "We're big-busted women, and we know how to dance."

On Christmas Day, when my sister, Dana, and I watched *Little Women*, I most enjoyed following Jo's quest to become a writer, scenes of her sitting at her attic desk near the frosty window late at night. As she dabbed pen into inkwell and scribbled away, something ignited inside of me. Possibility.

Because writers were nonexistent in our blue-collar Chicago neighborhood, saying I wanted to be one was like saying I wanted to be a princess. But watching *Little Women* was like getting permission to pursue the impossible.

I spent my childhood evenings scrawling in my diary and poring over books by flashlight. I wrote the title of my first novel in a "Book about Me" that I filled out in second grade. Under ideal profession, I wrote: "Writer," then, "My first novel will be called *Prisoner of Fate*."

Of course, I knew nothing about fate at that age—I wouldn't know for another twenty years. And so, in my opinion, the most horrifying moment in *Little Women* was not the father being wounded in the Civil War, or the death of young Beth, but when Amy burns all of Jo's manuscript pages in the fireplace out of spite. Back when "loss" was an abstract term, this seemed the absolute worst calamity one could endure.

Like Jo, who pursued her writing career in New York, I imagined that I would go off on my own and chase my dreams in the big city. I always envisioned living on the north side of Chicago after getting my master's, spending my days at coffee shops, sipping caramel lattes and typing away in the glow of my computer screen.

My visions of the future never revealed a man or children, and there was a quote in *Little Women* that I always identified with: "You are the gull, Jo, strong and wild, fond of the storm and the wind, flying far out to sea, and happy all alone."

I saw this as the way of writers. They were too self-involved to tend to others. Plus, life as a mother seemed so much harder than that of a career woman.

How selfless one had to be.

My favorite part of the *Little Women* movie was the arrival of a different sort of bundle—the pages of Jo's novel typeset by the publisher and bound in twine. This, I thought, was the greatest creation one could birth.

I spent my grad school years exactly as I had envisioned—working and pursuing writing in Chicago. During the week, I studied at Columbia College in the South Loop, then I passed the weekends at Panera or Starbucks in a writing frenzy fueled by espresso. It was my utopia.

Until Jamie entered my life.

He was from Massachusetts and we met while we were both on vacation in Florida. Our long-distance relationship began, and my whole world changed.

I moved into my own studio apartment in Chicago where Jamie would stay with me when he visited. I still spent Saturdays at cafés, but now I stared at his face instead of a Word document. When he went back to Boston, my bed felt so empty that my fantasy of living alone surrounded by books in a city high-rise now seemed like the loneliest form of existence.

During that time, I went out for Indian food with an office-mate and gushed about my latest decision to move to Massachusetts for Jamie. Still single in her 50s, my coworker encouraged me to publish before settling down and procreating. "Anyone can get pregnant," she said, "but not everyone can write a book."

It turns out the first part of her statement wasn't true. Not when the man has had testicular cancer and the chemo has affected the speed of his sperm. Not when the woman has undiagnosed hypothyroidism, hindering ovulation.

At twenty-four, I moved East and Jamie proposed to me. I traded my *Poets and Writers* magazines for *Modern Bride*. At the age of twenty-six, we moved to the rural burbs of Massachusetts. Just before I turned twenty-seven, I married Jamie, and at twenty-eight, we started operation pregnancy. What prompted me to choose a life so different from the one I had originally imagined? Maybe it was my innate desire to always pursue life's next steps. Or maybe it was that family Christmas scene from *Little Women* I was after—the colonial house, the fireplace, a living room filled with laughter.

Built in 1907, the house that Jamie and I bought just before we got married possessed a warm, antiquated appeal. Exposed wood beams ribbed the ceiling of the living room; a cast-iron stove heated the first floor. The second level boasted a small room so ideal for a little boy that I could imagine our future son doing his homework at the built-in desk. I could see his wooden trains on the shelves and his bed under the skylight, the stars singing him to sleep.

A year into our marriage, Jamie and I attempted our first in-vitro fertilization cycle, and after a month of hormones, I was ripe with egg follicles. I resembled the women my cousins and I had once imitated—curvy and voluptuous, albeit a bit bloated. Each of my ovaries grew from the size of grapes to what felt like grapefruits, and my eggs were ready to be harvested.

The retrieval was a quick outpatient procedure. The doctor went through my cervix and extracted my eggs via a needlelike syringe. The retrieval only took about fifteen minutes and after I came to, we were free to go. We were in and out of the clinic in under two hours.

It all seemed so effortless, so painless.

The nurses told me to go home and rest. I didn't have to lie in bed all day; I just needed to stay hydrated and avoid strenuous activity.

When we emerged from the clinic, the fall landscape blazed orange and red.

We drove down the back roads, the tires kicking up crunchy leaves in our wake. Jamie drummed the steering wheel while I rolled down the window and inhaled the crisp air.

"Three days," I said, "and we'll have a baby in here."

I rubbed my stomach, and Jamie placed his hand on top of mine.

"Three days," he said.

I was feeling so good that, as we drove through Concord, I asked Jamie to stop at Orchard House. Because I had canceled my university classes for the procedure, we now had the entire Tuesday to spend together—a rarity I wanted to take advantage of. True, the doctors had said to "take it easy," but to me, that meant not climbing any mountains or running any marathons. A little house tour wouldn't hurt anybody.

Jamie and I passed the time until the next tour by perusing the gift shop on the lower level. But as I blissfully looked at old rocking chairs and photographs of the Alcott family—items meant to turn back time—my own hourglass was losing sand much too quickly. Because of the sharp syringe used to extract my eggs, my ovaries were like water balloons with dozens of pinpricks. My right ovary had clotted on its own, but, unbeknownst to me, my left ovary hadn't. It gushed blood that drowned my organs as I flipped through Louisa's books in the gift shop. I can imagine the two halves of my body fighting—my left ovary versus my right—my desire for independence versus my longing for motherhood.

Did I intensify the bleeding by climbing the steep stairs from the parlor to the bedrooms? Would it have clotted if I hadn't walked around for the full hour of the tour, if I hadn't stopped to admire the four-post beds, the desk where Louisa wrote her novels? Would I have saved myself from emergency surgery, a grueling recovery, depression, marital strain, and a failed pregnancy attempt if I had just gone home that day?

Or was this my fate?

PART I

Chapter

1

used to love waking up with Chicago. I loved knowing my route, walking quickly, carrying a heavy bag, changing from gym shoes to high heels and back again.

Before I met Jamie, before I lived in my studio apartment, I lived with my parents while I studied and worked in the city. Every morning, I sat in the same Metra car, in the same seat, by the same window. As the train hummed toward the city, I put on my makeup and sipped my coffee. I cherished the shared quietness of the other riders, loved seeing the same woman organize her purse every day and the same man read the *Chicago Tribune* in his ritualistic order. This was my family. These were my people.

When the train pulled into its depot, we herded out the door and onto the platform, then up the escalator and past the newsstand. Inside Union Station, we smelled the ammonia of mopped floors, the coffee brewing, the bagels being toasted. At the doors, we braced ourselves for the chill of the fall morning, tasted the metallic city oxygen on our tongues. We crossed the Jackson Bridge over the Chicago River and passed the hunched man selling the *Streetwise* newspaper.

We moved silently but efficiently, waking up with every step. We shifted our bags up our shoulders, then stepped out into traffic, dodging bikers and cars. We raced the L trains, the bikes, the buses, and the cabs to prove we could arrive to work before them. We were warriors of the city.

By the time I arrived at the Tribune Tower each morning for my internship at *Chicago* magazine, my cheeks were cold but rosy, my eyes wind-dried but awake.

I was alive.

And, at the time, I thought this was all I needed: My city. My people.

Chicago had everything—skyscrapers, jogging paths, coffee shops, restaurants, beaches. My family had moved from the South Side to a suburb right outside the city. Dana would be going to college less than an hour away. Every single one of my friends lived in Chicago. I was broke, but my life was rich. I hung out at Katy's South Loop apartment on Friday afternoons, went barhopping in Lincoln Park with Courtney on Saturday nights, jogged by the lake with Jenny on Sunday mornings. And I was sure that Chicago had a husband for me, too—a well-dressed, well-read North-sider like the one I searched for over cocktails. I just hadn't found him yet.

Then, while on a trip to Florida with Mom, I did find him. There was just one little catch: he wasn't from Chicago.

Mom and I were sitting on a sunny restaurant patio, and as I anticipated returning to the hotel for a relaxing night, Mom said, "Let's go out!"

I eyed her empty cocktail glass. She rarely drank, and I wasn't sure what to expect from her if we went to the bars together.

"Don't be such an old lady," she said and shooed at me with her hand, as if I were the forty-one-year-old and she the grad student.

Ever since the plane had touched down in Tampa, she'd

been treating me more as a friend than a daughter, as if we were on spring break together. In fact, with her petite build and long hair, Mom could pass for a college coed upon first glance. But up close, her sunken eyes revealed the weight of the other roles she'd played—a wife at eighteen, a mother at nineteen, a divorcée at twenty, a new wife at twenty-two, a second-time mom at twenty-four.

Dad and Dana hadn't come to Florida because of Dana's soccer tournament. Though Dad was technically my stepdad and Dana my half sister, they'd always been my family, and I thought about what we'd be doing if they were here with us. We'd probably be talking about going back to the hotel pool instead of discussing my unsuccessful dating life. It was fun to laugh with Mom about my string of failed relationships—the most recent being with Andrew the Alcoholic who'd drunkenly pissed the bed one too many times—but it felt odd too, to be confiding in her like she was my sorority sister rather than my mother.

When we got into a taxi, Mom asked the driver where the nightlife was, and he dropped us off at the Green Iguana in Ybor City. Jimmy Buffett songs hovered in the humid night air as we paid our cab fare and lined up by the doorman. Inside, we squeezed our way through the sweaty mob and Mom decided to be my wing-woman, shouting, "How 'bout that guy? What about that tall one over there?"

The band played "It's Five O'Clock Somewhere" and we claimed our space at the thatched-roof bar. Mom swatted my hand when I ordered our drinks. "That's what they're here for," she said, nodding at the men next to us.

"Mom," I said, laughing. "I can buy my own beer."

She brought a Marlboro Light to her lips and lit it. "I'm just saying," she said, exhaling smoke, "you look nice." She gestured toward my flowy skirt, the sun streaks in my hair. "Why not take advantage?"

I paid the bartender and handed Mom her Long Island iced tea. "It's OK, Ma," I said, teasing. "You can calm down there, cupid."

The beer and music loosened me up a little. It was April and Chicago's snowy streets seemed like another universe. I'd left my winter boots and schoolwork at home, replacing them with a tan and smile. Here, the bar air smelled like piña coladas, and I settled onto my stool.

Mom looked past the crowd toward the open windows where twinkle lights lined the streets and young people walked in packs. Something about the Florida night made her nostalgic, and she reminisced about when she and Dad had first met.

"He was in great shape back then," she said, shaking her head. Her voice trailed off, but I knew all the ways that Mom and Dad had changed since meeting, how they'd betrayed each other, how they'd sought solace in their various vices—Dad in food, Mom in nicotine.

Mom took a long drag off her cigarette and squinted. It was evident, all the things she was pondering. *What happened to my life? When did I stop having fun?*

I was asking myself questions, too, like: *Am I too screwed up to fall in love? If I do, will it be just as messy as their marriage?*

A cherry stem lay on Mom's napkin and I knotted it around my finger, feeling equally twisted between wanting to be her confidant and wanting to be her daughter. That night was the first glimpse I'd ever gotten of younger Mom, of the Bonnie who would have existed if life hadn't gotten so complicated. I wanted to hug her for all the fun she'd missed out on while she'd been changing diapers and cleaning house. At the same time, I wanted to convince her and Dad to seek counseling so that I didn't have to bear the heaviness of their hurt anymore.

I finished my beer, and tried to order another, but the bartenders were buried, barely able to keep up with the crowd that pressed against the counter. That's when Mom tapped the guy next to me on the shoulder.

In one swift move, she pointed at me, and said, "How about buying my daughter a drink?"

He turned toward us, not sure if he'd heard her right, then laughed as I said, "Apparently she thinks I'm not capable of getting it myself."

But Mom wasn't done embarrassing me. "You're just her type," she told him.

In some ways she was right. He was blonde and broad-shouldered, older looking than the scrawny twentysomethings that saturated the Chicago bar scene.

Without missing a beat, he extended his hand and said, "I'm Jamie. What would you like to drink?"

While Mom chatted with his friend, Jamie and I took our beers to a high-top table and talked.

I learned that Jamie preferred T-shirts to ties, movies to books. He was a former chef ten years my senior, and he lived in a suburb of Boston where he worked as a project manager at a signage company. Because it seemed so unlikely that two people from two different states could form a budding romance at a tourist bar, there was no pressure, and we felt instantly comfortable around each other.

The live band played their last Buffett song and the lights dimmed, noting the change from Margaritaville to nightclub. When a '90s tune came on, the crowd cheered, forming a mass of bouncing bodies.

Mom swayed her hips, and a guy danced near her. *Will he notice the wedding ring on her finger?* I wondered. *Will it even make a difference to him?*

I peeled the label off my beer, contemplating whether to intervene.

Jamie felt the heaviness of my thoughts and pulled me over

to him, hugging me hard. It was the sort of hug I'd expect from a serious boyfriend—a long, secure hold. It was exactly what I needed to realize that Mom was her own person, that it wasn't my job to be her parent. It was my turn to be twenty-two.

So I danced, performing the running man, the butterfly, *and* the tootsie roll back-to-back. In the humid bar, a sweaty Jamie laughed and clapped for me. I curtsied. Then, in an instinctive gesture, I wiped the sweat off of his forehead. It was a simple thing, the sort of thing a wife might do, and it charmed him. I saw it happen. I saw his brain calibrate and his attention hone in on me.

He leaned against the high-top, and I asked him what he liked to do for fun. He described his parents' cabin in Maine, how they grilled and sat around the fire. Jamie seemed a rare species to me. I waited for him to do what Chicago guys did: name-drop, spin stories about his amazing life. But his every movement was calm, sincere—the way he stood in the same spot like he had nowhere better to be, the way he tilted his head when he listened to me. His stillness in a crowd of rowdy barflies was so captivating that I asked if I could kiss him. He smiled and straightened up, waiting for my hands to cup his face.

When he asked for my number, I gave it to him, hoping that he'd call me when he got back to Massachusetts, though I didn't think about how we'd sustain a relationship while living eight hundred miles apart.

After I got home from Florida, Jamie mailed me a letter—an actual handwritten letter. "There's something intriguing about you," he wrote. "You're always on my mind."

We talked on the phone for hours every night over the next three months, then I bought a ticket to visit him.

During my plane ride to Massachusetts, only one thought occupied my mind: *What the hell am I doing?*

At Logan Airport, as I trudged toward baggage claim, the thought persisted, accompanied by: *What if we HATE each other?*

Yes, we'd bonded during our nightly phone conversations, but that didn't guarantee anything.

We'd planned to spend five days together. That meant that if we despised each other, we still had almost a week of suffering through beach walks and car rides. And what about the sleeping arrangements?

As the escalator carried me down to the airport's lower level, I couldn't even look into the crowd of expectant eyes and wide smiles because I was so terrified that I would overlook Jamie. What if I didn't recognize him, and he was standing right in front of me? How bad would it be if I walked right past him and kept on searching for the man I thought I had met in Florida? So I called his cell phone. If he stood amongst the group, I would see him reach into his pocket and put the phone to his ear. I would know it was him. A great idea, except that no cell phones rang and no one reached into their pockets.

What if Jamie had chickened out and decided not to come? Would he actually do that? What if I had to go back to Chicago and admit that I had made a mistake, that my instincts had been wrong?

At the baggage belt, I waited for my suitcase and considered checking the list of return flights. Among the emerging luggage, my bag still hadn't appeared, so I stared at the circling suitcases. Then, I smelled the familiar, woodsy cologne Jamie had worn in Florida and felt a tap on my right shoulder. It was him. It was him. It was him. The air disappeared from my lungs and hives crawled up my chest. Somehow I managed to pivot on my heel and face him. Same blonde hair, same calm stance, but I had been studying Jamie's picture for so long, it was a shock to see him as a fleshed-out human being. He wore a simple red button-down and jeans. My skirt and wedges seemed too dressy.

Here we were looking at each other—the moment we'd been eagerly awaiting—and I had no idea what to say. It was as if those three months of talking had disappeared. So I spurted out the only thing I could come up with.

"Are you hungry?" I asked as I rummaged through my purse for my stale airline pretzels. "I have some snacks."

He laughed at me, a loud bellow, then smiled crookedly.

"Come here, sweet girl," he said.

I stopped my search for the pretzels and let him envelop me in a warm hug, which was exactly as I remembered from Tampa—tight and secure and safe and passionate and vulnerably close. I squeezed him back and felt my heartbeat racing, while his thumped slowly and steadily against mine. In his presence, all the questions slipped from my mind. We were going to get along just fine.

A few months into our long-distance relationship, we visited his parents' Maine cabin and went for our first hike together.

Jamie traversed the trails slowly. He stopped often to ponder an animal track, to watch a hawk hover in the sky. Jamie's close-together eyes and sharp nose resembled the very bird he observed.

I charged ahead and gripped tree branches to help me up the rocky terrain. My shoes hopped from one spot to another, while Jamie's made deep ditches in the dirt. Examining our tracks in the mud, I wondered how his firm footprints and my frantic ones could reach the same peak.

But, somehow, they did.

Back at the cabin, I ran out to the lake and cannonballed into the water. Jamie stayed on the dock and sat in an Adirondack chair under the shade of a tree. He took in the landscape that I didn't see because I was too busy chopping my hand through the waves and taking rapid breaths. Back and forth I swam, counting laps, switching from breaststroke to back. The cold water pumped my blood. Jamie leaned back in his chair and looked out at the trees and the mountains. He inhaled. Deeply. Treading water, I followed his gaze to the canoe across the lake, the hovering hawk. I slowed my treading and took it all in—the water lapping against a rock, the bark shedding off a birch tree.

I realized, in that moment, that Jamie was the only person who had ever clicked my world into focus.

So, I climbed onto the dock, wrapped myself in a towel, and sat in the chair with him.

That afternoon, we watched the world together.

Something happened to me during this time. I became a compulsive hand holder, a head rubber, a public kisser, a lap sitter, a phone talker.

One needn't look any farther than Jamie's nightstand to find proof of my love. Over the two years we dated long distance, Jamie's drawers filled with my letters, ticket stubs, mixed CDs, photos.

Too strapped to buy cards, I drew him ones—a Thanksgiving turkey that looked like a dinosaur, a stick-figure couple having sex. Though I had given myself a weekly twenty-five dollar spending budget, I'd save and save so that when Jamie came to Chicago, I could treat him to a concert at the House of Blues or dinners atop the Hancock. The novel chapters I wrote in grad school were thinly fictionalized scenes of our relationship. I'd spend hours crafting each page and then send them to Jamie when I was done. They were the greatest love notes I could ever compose.

Jamie spoiled me too, but better than any weekend get-away on Nantucket was the gift of his home-cooked meals. I had been a simple eater, but with him, I ate pecan-crusted salmon and garlic cheddar mashed potatoes.

"You've got to taste this," he'd say, bringing a steaming forkful to my mouth.

Jamie made me want to consume every morsel of life. He made me want to stop, sit, notice, eat, hug, love. He made me want to pause.

And I did. In fact, I paused completely. The day after I graduated, I stopped living in Chicago and moved to Massachusetts for him.

Chapter

2

Our first winter together was magical. We were newly engaged. We didn't care that our rental house was less than eight hundred square feet, that our table took up our entire kitchen, that our washer-dryer acted as our pot rack. We didn't care that we had to run the faucet to keep the pipes from freezing, that the draft from the thin windows left us shivering. We didn't care that we had to duck every time we climbed our steep stairs, that our bedroom was really an attic with no closets, that the sloped ceilings prevented Jamie from standing straight.

My meager adjunct's salary at Framingham State University, our tight budget—none of it bothered us, because we kept each other warm that winter. Jamie made us chai tea lattes every morning. I scrambled eggs. I lined our front hallway with pictures of us, pictures of our new dog Tessa, pictures of Massachusetts, pictures of Maine. We spent entire Saturdays cuddled up on the couch in our fleece pajamas. In the afternoon, Jamie cooked hearty chili, eggplant soup. Then we layered up in mismatched winter gear and held gloved hands for our walks in the woods with Tessa. We threw sticks for her and held our arms out like mummies, marching toward her until she wagged her tail and sprinted in circles. We explored different trails, paused to consider the species of a tree.

After our hikes, we got cheap takeout and drove home admiring the Christmas lights. The three of us snuggled up on the couch and used pillows on our laps as dinner trays. Tessa lay against me while I lay against Jamie, and we watched movies. Around midnight, Jamie and I headed up to our cold bedroom. We made love under layers of blankets. We fogged up the windows.

On my first birthday away from home, I awoke, selfishly expecting to smell a cake baking and see banners hanging on every wall, the way I had growing up. Mom and Dad had always made a big deal over my birthday, decorating the whole house in the middle of the night so I'd wake up to a celebration. But here, Jamie and Tessa snored next to me in the dim light of the morning.

When I stepped out of the shower, Jamie was stretching in the doorway. He hugged me and wished me a happy birthday, and I squeezed him back but had to turn my face so that he wouldn't see my disappointment. The entire time I blow-dried my hair, I waited for him to slide a card or gift onto the bathroom counter, but Jamie fed Tessa and went about his usual morning routine.

During my ride to the university and the whole time I taught my English classes, I brooded over the lack of thought that had gone into my day. *I moved all the way across the country for him,* I thought, *and he can't even hang a banner?*

That afternoon, homesickness rode home with me down 495, making me taste the chocolate frosting that Dad had always put on my cake, the vanilla ice cream that Mom had always served alongside it.

Even my yoga class did nothing to calm me, and by the time I got home, I was gritting my teeth. I parked in our gravel drive and stayed in my car for a minute, searching the windows for any sign of streamers but found none. I was being ridiculous, but my resentment still mounted.

When I walked up the front stairs carrying my heavy workbag, I heard a rustling inside. Then, I opened the door, and on cue, "They Say It's Your Birthday" blared through the speakers. Jamie and Tessa popped into the hallway wearing party hats. While Tessa pawed at her hat, Jamie blew a horn and sang to me.

"Go kiss the mamas," he told Tessa.

Banners and balloons lined our hallway and Tessa stared at them, at us, trying to figure out what the hell we crazy humans were up to. When I crouched down and rubbed her neck, she licked my cheek.

Using his best Tessa voice, Jamie said, "Mamas, you're amazing."

We laughed and Jamie pulled me up for a hug. This time, my squeeze back was genuine. He led me into the kitchen, where a chocolate cake awaited me, as did a gift certificate to a salon—a luxury he knew I wouldn't splurge on for myself.

That night, we ate cake together on the couch, exchanging chocolaty kisses, and I felt wonderfully, decadently full.

Visitors always felt like burdens, like people crashing our honeymoon. When Katy came to Boston, I neglected her so that I could go for walks with Jamie and Tessa. When Courtney and Marie visited, I drove them around our quiet suburb, and Courtney asked if I missed the city. I shook my head and explained that life was so much simpler and quieter out here. The people were so much nicer. She tilted her head at me in a way that meant *Cut the bullshit,* and I had to turn away from her gaze, afraid she'd see right through me.

At our house, Courtney paused in the hallway to look at the photos I'd hung. Her face tightened.

"Where are all your pictures of us?" she asked. I scanned the framed photos ready to defend myself, but there was no evidence of my Chicago life. All of those pictures were in crates in our basement, as were the photos of my family.

It was especially hard to look at photos of Mom. She hadn't been ecstatic about me moving away. When Jamie had proposed to me, Mom said that he was trying to steal me away from her, from my family.

"He's playing you like a violin," she told me during one of our many phone fights. "Why couldn't he move to Chicago for you?" she asked.

"He tried," I said. "He couldn't find a job."

She exhaled, and I knew she was smoking in the garage.

"He couldn't find a job in Chicago," she hissed, "or he didn't want to?"

"Please just be happy for me."

"I hope you'll never have to experience what it's like for your child to walk out on you," she said. Then she added, "You think it's just that easy, Nadine? You meet some guy and get married? It's more complicated than that."

But in Massachusetts, life was so much easier, so much happier, and I started to think that maybe I had left my complications behind in Chicago.

I'd get off of the phone and complain to Jamie that Mom was projecting all of her unhappiness onto me.

"It's not my fault she's miserable," I said.

But sometimes I felt that it was my fault. If she hadn't had me, she might have gone to college, traveled more. She would have easily divorced my father without the complexity of me in the equation, and she would have met Dad at a time when she was free, not burdened with a baby. She and Dad would have remained giddy-in-love.

But that wasn't the reality, and I'd witnessed many screaming matches between them. Their fights were loud, explosive, full of fingers in faces and fiery insults. But just as fiercely as they could yell, they could laugh. I guessed it was why they were still together decades later despite their resentment—they were able to poke fun at each other.

Jamie's parents had thirty-five years of marriage under their belt, and early on, I asked Jamie what bonded them.

"I've never heard them argue," he said.

"Never?" I asked, disbelieving.

"Never."

Every time I saw Jamie's parents, they'd be sitting together, fingers intertwined. It was like seeing a rare exhibit at a museum.

Jamie's mom was a hugger, a baker, a sitter, a knitter. Mom was a coffee drinker, a chain-smoker, an aerobics instructor. But despite Mom's unaffectionate nature, she'd been an active parent—played board games with us, somersaulted in the pool with us. She had taken us roller-skating and bowling, sledding and skiing.

In Massachusetts, when I thought of these moments, I yearned for her. I left Jamie and Tessa at home and went for long jogs alone. My legs sprinted up hills while my mind analyzed my relationship with Mom. *Why can't she just tell me she misses me?* I wondered.

I didn't ask myself why I couldn't tell her the same thing.

Because our relationship was so complex, it was easier not to talk. So I began ignoring Mom's calls.

I wasn't calling my sister much these days, either. Not because I didn't want to. Dana liked Jamie and supported my move, and I missed her, but I got so wrapped up with being in love that I rarely checked in to see how her semester was going.

At work one day, I met another adjunct instructor who was an alum of Dana's college. He asked what street Dana lived on, which sorority she had pledged. My cheeks blazed. I didn't know the answer to either question.

It seemed that as soon as I'd moved out East for Jamie, my brain had turned off Chicago like a switch. I convinced myself that I was a better person in Massachusetts. With Jamie and me in our little bubble, my soul felt pure and untainted. I reasoned that Chicago was too chaotic. My family was too loud and dysfunctional. My single city friends just didn't understand why I'd want to live in the burbs with my fiancé.

My brain could only process one emotion at a time. It couldn't be giddy-in-love and simultaneously miss the Midwest. So, I opted to bask in the happiness of Massachusetts and hoped that it would never wear off.

Chapter

3

Jamie and I got married in Maine on the same lake I had jumped into after our first hike together. It was a sunny August afternoon and the backdrop for our ceremony was the same outcropping of trees and mountains that Jamie and I had explored throughout our four years together.

As I waited to walk down the grassy aisle, a red fence separated me from all of the wedding guests, who sat in white chairs on the sprawling lawn overlooking the lake.

Jamie and I had picked the playlist, and I'd chosen "Making Plans" by Miranda Lambert for my bridesmaids' procession. Jamie had chosen Tom Petty's song "Here Comes My Girl" for my entrance. It felt fitting that we'd both picked songs referring to me as Jamie's girl, and despite my independent façade, I was so damn proud to be his.

When Tom Petty sang, "Watch her walk," the red gate opened, revealing the glittering lake and looming mountains. My bridesmaids' pale yellow gowns blew in the breeze while Jamie's groomsmen stood tall and proper. And there, at the tip of the peninsula, under the forsythia arbor, Jamie waited with a crooked smile, looking like this was the easiest decision he had ever made. With Dad on my left side and my father on my right, I walked under a bridge of willow trees and down the slope toward Jamie. There was something timeless about it all—my lace gown and blusher veil, Jamie's black tux—like we could have been a bride and groom from any era and would prevail during the decades to come.

A few feet from the arbor, I couldn't take it anymore, and I hopped toward Jamie. The guests clapped, and Jamie whispered in my ear, "You're beautiful."

When it was time for our declarations of love, the officiant gave me the microphone, and Dana handed me my notes along with a tissue, just in case. I smoothed my dress and cleared my throat.

"Jamie," I said. "I love you because you always have dinner waiting for me when I come home, and these are real meals, not the Lean Cuisines I used to make for myself. I love you because you stay in bed with me on Saturday mornings, like there is nowhere better to be. I love you because you sing in an embarrassingly high-pitched voice to '80s tunes."

Jamie shook his head in denial, and the guests laughed.

"I love you," I continued, "because whenever we go shopping, you always want to buy Tessa another dog bed, even though she already has three of them. I love you because you always hold my hand in the car. I love you because you have a strange phobia of lotion and the sticky feeling it leaves on your skin."

Jamie shuddered, jokingly, as if the mere idea of moisturizer was enough to make him gag.

I knew that my next few sentences would make me emotional, and I took a deep breath to keep my composure. "I love you because every time I see that handsome smile of yours, I get butterflies like a teenager in love. I love you because being with you in the worst of places is better than being in the most beautiful place alone. And," I said, looking up from my paper to Jamie, "I love you because you changed every bitter thought I ever had about love."

I dabbed my eyes with my tissue and handed the microphone to Jamie, but there was so much more I could have listed, like how handy he was, how he stripped carpet and installed ceiling fans. He was efficient, too. Whereas I deliberated over outfits every morning, wrestling through a pile of clothes I hadn't hung, Jamie put his deodorant on at exactly 6:50 and kept his keys in the same spot atop his dresser. How different we were, and yet our oppositeness had brought us here to this lakeside altar.

Jamie took his paper from his suit pocket and said, "Nadine, I want to share with everyone just a few of the reasons why I love you.

"I love your passion for teaching and your ambition. I love your positive attitude and how your nose wrinkles when you smile." He paused and looked at my geeky grin. "Like that," he said.

"I love how thoughtful you are. I love your courage and creativity. I love your dance moves."

I wiggled and shimmied as proof.

Jamie laughed into the microphone and added, "I love how you always ask me to tell you about my day. I love your natural instincts with children. I love how you always put me in my place when I need it."

I batted my eyes in a "who me?" motion and the guests laughed.

Jamie folded his paper, until just the last few lines were left, and said, "I love how you always leave me little notes and how you always tell me how proud you are of me. But most of all," he said, reaching for my hand, "I love the opportunity you have given me to call you my wife."

The profoundness of the moment caught me when Jamie said, "wife." *I* was his *wife.* Somehow over the course of the last four years, it had happened, the thing I thought I was the least capable of—love. I'd been able to love this man fully, wholly, and I'd openly accepted the love he'd given me. Now here we were, husband and wife.

After our kiss, we raised our clasped hands in cheer and said, "Cue the music." Then we walked into our future to the tune of Lindsey Buckingham's "It Was You."

Just a few months after Jamie and I exchanged vows, we decided it was time to talk about babies. Like most naive newlyweds, we thought that getting married and purchasing a home had somehow prepared us for parenthood. Unlike our tiny rental, our *Little Women* house was spacious and warm. It dripped with history. I could imagine its first owners nailing the wooden ceiling beams into place, sanding the shelves that lined the wall of our future child's room. True, we'd had to expand our search much farther from Boston to get something we could afford, so our home was in a remote rural suburb that was as sparse as Chicago was bustling, but I reasoned that this would make our offspring's upbringing even more wholesome.

We decided that I would stop taking my birth control during a trip to Chicago in January 2011. I was twenty-seven; Jamie was thirty-seven. We were sitting at my favorite bakery in Lincoln Park called Molly's Cupcakes, and as we licked frosting off our fingers, we talked about the upcoming year.

"Maybe we'll have a little addition to our family," Jamie said.

I scraped the last bit of cupcake off my plate and said, "I have a hunch that we'll have a boy."

This was a strange premonition because, growing up, I'd lived in a home dominated by females. Dana and I had even chosen a female Yorkshire terrier as a pet, so it didn't make any sense that my subconscious craved a boy. It had everything to do with the picture—the framed one of Jamie as a toddler that sat on our windowsill. I imagined our son to look exactly like Jamie did in the photo. His curly locks were almost as light as his skin. His distinct nose was already starting to protrude. He was just sitting—not running, not babbling—just sitting, dangling his chunky legs, and smiling. He was so young and already so aware of the most important thing in life: the pause.

I imagined myself holding this boy, this replica of Jamie. I was sure that this being would make me be my best self. His laughter would make me stand still. His smile would be enough to halt me in my constant desire to be better, to seek out the next thing, to go to the next place, to accomplish the next task. We would spend afternoons stacking blocks, reading books, singing songs, or simply rocking in a glider.

In these visions of me holding our son, I had a chance to start over and erase my flaws. I wouldn't be guarded. I wouldn't be defensive. This baby wouldn't have to know my past—like when I was an angsty preteen babysitting Dana and I slapped her hard, or how I starved and binged in high school, how I drank way too much in college, blacked out often, put myself in compromising positions, landed on academic probation, how I'd strung along my college boyfriend after I knew it was over, how, at twenty-one, I flirted with a married man and hoped he'd leave his wife for me.

This baby would erase every negative trait. I could reform myself. I'd become more involved in Dana's life, hang my friends' pictures up on my walls, maybe even reconnect with Mom.

Recently, I'd gone from avoiding some of Mom's calls to ignoring all of them.

During our last argument, Mom had said, "What about me? Do you have any idea how this is affecting me?"

"I'm so fucking sick of hearing about you," I'd told her, and hung up the phone.

Mom had been shouting "What about me?" for as long as I could remember and maybe even before then, when she was twenty, recently divorced, and raising me on a Honolulu Marine base she'd moved to for my father. Maybe there was a time when she was satisfied, like when she met Dad and they were inseparable—evident from pictures of their early days stealing smooches on Kailua Beach while I crawled around in the sand, sunburned and potbellied in my floral bikini. But then they moved to Mom's hometown of Chicago, got married, bought a house, had Dana, and our home was filled with Mom's rages, constant complaints of being broke.

When I was fourteen, we moved to the suburbs. Mom stopped working at the bank and became a personal trainer, then a masseuse. It always seemed, though, that Mom was slipping away, seeking a private moment, whether it was into the garage for a cigarette or off to get coffee. When she scrubbed dishes, she yelled at the air, "What about what I need?"

As a teen, I had a love-hate relationship with her. When we weren't tight on money, we went shopping at Kohl's and got Frappuccinos at Starbucks. We worked out together, silently competing to have the better abs, the leaner legs. But when we weren't friends, we were enemies, and our fights sometimes resulted in Mom pulling my hair, scratching me with her nails. Her favorite saying was, "I brought you into this world, and I can take you back out." I held up my hand, threatened to hit her. I yelled that I hated her. After our fights, I'd write her a note explaining my side of the argument. My signatures ended with forced apologies. Mom would smoke in the garage and ignore my presence for a few days, then we'd be back to picking out cute outfits and bonding over java, not a word mentioned about the fight.

During Mom's rants about my move to Massachusetts, I stopped writing apology letters. *Why should I say I'm sorry?* I wondered. *What's so terrible about moving in with the man I love?*

I stopped responding when she listed her grievances—how I hadn't called her first thing on Mother's Day last year, how I hadn't involved her in my wedding planning. She had valid points, but I didn't want to hear them anymore.

Most recently, I'd expressed the hurt that I'd been carrying with me since childhood, and again, I'd heard, "What about me?" So I decided to stop talking to her.

Though she called me many times after that, I never picked up and never called her back.

I reasoned that, maybe, when Jamie and I had a child, I'd get the chance to be everything that Mom hadn't been to me.

At Molly's Cupcakes, Jamie placed our plates into the dish bin and we buttoned our coats. I grabbed my purse—my birth control nestled in the pocket—and it felt lighter with the knowledge that I wouldn't be taking those pink pills anymore. We left the bakery holding hands and entered the January afternoon feeling like anything was possible.

Chapter

4

We decided to name our baby Veal.

Jamie and I came up with the moniker while walking Tessa just a couple days before heading to Europe. Our budget had been too tight after our wedding to take a real trip, so we'd saved up all year for this belated honeymoon. Our giddiness made the May afternoon warmer, our steps lighter. Feeding off of our bliss, Tessa leapt down the trail like a floppy-eared deer.

"What if I get knocked up in Italy?" I joked as I hurled a stick into the woods and Tessa chased it.

Ever since I'd gone off of birth control five months ago, I'd been gaining weight and losing my hair. Then I'd started missing my periods. After months of being misdiagnosed with depression and "getting older," my doctor discovered my hypothyroidism. But now that I was taking thyroid pills, my cycles were supposed to be more regular, my hormones more controlled. If my new medicine worked its magic, I'd be ovulating—and getting pregnant—on the third day of our vacation. We knew from a recent semen analysis that, because of the chemo Jamie had received for his testicular cancer, some of his sperm swam slowly and in the wrong direction. But we'd known plenty of couples who had conceived after cancer, and we were going to be one of them. We just needed one strong swimmer.

Plus, I couldn't turn off the desire for motherhood. Over the last few months, the absence of our imagined son, the lack of him, had begun to show itself. The more I missed city life and my Chicago network, the more I longed for our child. Our bed seemed too big, our house too quiet. Every time I passed our second bedroom, I noted the daybed under the skylight where his crib should be, my files in the drawers where his clothes should reside. On my way to the bathroom in the morning, I expected to step on a rogue toy truck. I'd do dishes and hear a specific tinkling of water that resembled a child's laughter. I'd finish stacking the plates on a dish towel, turn off the faucet, and think *Where is he? Where's he hiding?* But only the silence answered. During the rare times we went out into our large backyard, I noticed the emptiness of a patio that didn't contain his baseball glove and bicycle. Despite the May heat wave, the winter cover remained on our pool because it didn't make sense to take it off if our child wouldn't be swimming in it. During hikes in the woods, my back felt too light. It seemed that without the weight of our son riding piggyback, I might just float away.

So, instead of telling Jamie that my very existence depended on a child that did not exist, I joked about Italian baby names. I told him that we'd have to name our child Bellagio or Maggiore after the location of its conception. Jamie teased that, instead, we should get our inspiration from Italian food, like formaggio or pesce. He scanned his brain for menu items he had cooked during his days as sous chef for The Florentina.

"How about Vitello Parmigiano?" he said, and we laughed and laughed just imagining our freckled, towheaded child having such a name. How fitting it was, too, that if our little veal looked anything like me during infancy, he would even resemble a baby cow—disproportioned and awkward.

In Italy, we discussed Vitello's upbringing as we snapped pictures of the Romeo and Juliet balcony in Verona and ate gelato in Sirmione. We uttered the name Vitello so much during our week abroad that when Jamie and I walked down the streets of Rome, I could almost feel our toddler's hand reaching up for mine. When we dined at cafés, my fork and knife instinctively cut my prosciutto into small pieces that I yearned to place onto our son's plate.

"To Vitello," I said when Jamie clinked my wine glass.

"To Vitello," Jamie said, smiling.

On Isola dei Pescatori—Fisherman's Island—I approached an embroidery booth and scanned the board of aprons and handkerchiefs. I pointed to a small bib. When I asked the seamstress to sew the word "Vitello" onto it with blue thread, she nodded, but her pupils laughed at us. She thought we didn't know that it meant "veal."

I fantasized that when we returned to the States and confirmed my pregnancy, I'd wrap the Vitello bib in a little blue box for my in-laws. They'd open it, assuming it a souvenir, but they'd soon find that it was an early birth announcement for their first grandchild. Since Jamie's official name was George James Johnstone IV, our son would be George James Johnstone V—the V standing, of course, for the fifth, but also, secretly, for Vitello.

I took a pregnancy test as soon as we landed in Massachusetts and swore, unwaveringly, that if our love hadn't created a baby, then our telekinetic wishes surely had.

But only one blue line appeared.

"Next month," we said as we stood in the bathroom looking at the plastic wand on the sink. "It will happen next month." But Jamie headed for the living room to pretend to watch TV, and I climbed upstairs to pretend to read, each of us silently missing the son that had lived only in our imaginations. That night, our house felt barren.

With each new page on the calendar, with each single line on my Clear Blue Easy tests, the Vitello bib haunted me more. I moved it from the top of my dresser to my underwear drawer, then folded it under a stack of bras, and finally wrapped it in a camisole so that the embroidered letters couldn't remind me of the child we didn't have.

In Italy, I thought that because we had given our unborn baby a nickname and had even chosen his gender through the blue thread on the bib, we would automatically conceive him. I had believed—in my young naïveté—that we were above health conditions, fertility percentages, and fate.

But there was so, so much we didn't know.

Chapter

5

n July, I still wasn't getting regular periods. When they did come, I hurled the box of tampons across the bathroom. Becoming ever more baby obsessed, I took my temperature and peed on ovulation sticks every morning. I came on to Jamie every night, but he could sense that my mission was pregnancy, not pleasure. Our intimate moments began to feel like a chore.

The thyroid medicine and the eating well had done nothing for my cycles or my physical appearance. On my petite frame, my recent fifteen-pound weight gain left me unable to fit into my clothes. Add to that some bulbous acne, and I'd never felt more unattractive.

When my periods still didn't regulate and my waist didn't slim, my ob-gyn ran more tests and discovered high prolactin levels. I had to undergo an MRI to see if a pituitary tumor lurked in my brain. The MRI images revealed no growths, yet my levels remained high. The doctor told me that, usually, prolactin hormone production only increases during pregnancy, and, among other things, prepares the breasts for lactation.

Remembering a grad school friend with a similar problem,

I cringed. Her rising prolactin caused her to spurt milk whenever her partner caressed her chest. What if the next time Jamie and I fooled around, my body rewarded him with a mouthful of milk?

I received no explanations for my prolactinoma, only that it affected the yield of thyroid hormones, which is why I had hypothyroidism and why my symptoms weren't disappearing even though I took my medicine diligently. And, I was told, the estrogen in my birth control had previously controlled the prolactin, which is why these issues materialized only after I had stopped taking the pill.

Why hadn't anyone brought this up when my hypothyroidism was discovered? Why had it taken three months and ten trips to the blood lab to uncover this?

The doctor called in a prescription for prolactin medicine, which instantly regulated my cycle to twenty-eight days.

The next time I ovulated, I made sex our sole mission, but two weeks later, my period came, its cramps announcing that we were yet again without child.

My gynecologist said that she usually encourages the average couple to try conceiving for a year before considering IVF. It had only been eight months since that January day we'd decided that I should get off of birth control, and my hormone imbalance had made conception virtually impossible. So I debated if we should keep trying on our own now that my cycles were regular. But eight months feels like eight years when you're waiting to get pregnant. An acquaintance had conceived a son around the same time I'd gone off of birth control, and she was due to deliver next month. If I were like her and the many couples who get pregnant right away, I'd be packing my hospital bag and readying the nursery. But we weren't one of those lucky couples; we weren't even one of those average couples.

We already knew we were contending with compromised sperm. But maybe below-average motility and morphology were actually detrimental to conception. Because the urologist Jamie had seen for the analysis wasn't a reproductive expert and hadn't given a concrete prediction about our fertility chances, I decided it was time for us to see someone who could give us answers. So I got a referral and talked to a representative at a fertility clinic who ensured me that, based on Jamie's results, we had every right to seek assistance. She scheduled an appointment for the following week so we could discuss our options with a specialist.

I circled the date on our calendar and wrote "appointment," but I really wanted to write "we're going to have a baby," because, to me, this appointment meant that the possibility of a baby could become a reality. This single appointment could change our lives forever.

I got to the clinic before Jamie, and the first thing I noticed was the lobby. It was empty. This was a makeshift satellite office forty miles from the city headquarters, and it looked as if someone had thrown everything together the day before. The sitting area consisted of two old chairs, and the chipped end table was covered with infertility pamphlets. Boxes, stacked and unpacked, lined a narrow hallway. The wall of the specialist's office was a big glass window lined with '80s venetian blinds. The thin glass did nothing to buffer our doctor's voice. For twenty minutes she complained—presumably into her cell phone—about somebody she was less than pleased with. She ranted about how inept this person was, said that when she got home, she was going to take her anger out on the tennis court. She was going to envision the ball as his head and "slam it to the ground."

Jamie walked into the lobby right then, and I thought for a second about grabbing his hand and saying, "Let's get the fuck out of here." But I stayed put in my uncomfortable seat. I did this sometimes when I was desperate or in foreign territory—I shushed my intuition—only to look back later and wonder why I hadn't listened to myself.

Jamie sat down next to me, and we feigned composure. We made fun of the depressing brochures, which showed women past prime reproductive age. The literature didn't address male infertility or our biggest fear: Even if the doctor forced Jamie's sperm and my egg together in a petri dish, were his sperm so affected that they still wouldn't fertilize my eggs? And then what? When void of children, what happens to a wife? A husband? A marriage?

Almost thirteen years ago, just before Jamie's tumor removal and chemo, the doctors had urged him to store some of his semen, so that if his cancer treatments made him sterile, he could use the sperm to fertilize an embryo. And he did store the sample—until he could no longer afford the monthly fees. It was six years before we met. He was in his mid-twenties, not thinking about marriage and babies, so he let his payments lapse, and his sample was discarded. Now, both he and I wondered if, all those years ago, he'd unknowingly thrown away our only chance at having biological children.

I'd once seen a documentary TV special that had followed infertile adults on their journey to become parents. One particular couple received results that revealed that the husband was completely sterile. The wife could barely look at her spouse. You could see that this woman simultaneously wanted to comfort her husband and file for divorce. Her dream of parenthood seemed to trump even the desire to stay committed to the man she loved.

At the time, I'd wondered how this could happen. How

could the yearning for something she'd never had be greater than the love of the partner she already had?

I wanted to believe that Jamie and I could overcome anything. But, instead, I saw quiet years stretching ahead—us doing all the things we'd always wanted to—buying an RV, traveling, opening up a little café that hosted writing and cooking classes. But I worried that my resentment would grow as my baby-bearing years slipped away from me.

These thoughts made me feel like a horrible person, and I imagined the roles reversing. What if my hormone imbalance hadn't been corrected with medicine? What if I was the one with incurable fertility problems? Would Jamie still stay with me? I knew he would. I also knew he would handle the resentment better than I could.

Finally, our doctor opened up the thin door, exposing her equally thin self.

"I'm sorry to keep you waiting," she said, as if she'd spent the last twenty minutes reading over our file and not ranting on the phone.

She led us into a large office that was empty minus her diplomas and a picture of a young boy.

We sat down, and she took a sip of her Diet Coke through a bendy straw.

"Is that your son?" I asked, pointing to the picture.

She smiled and nodded.

I couldn't help myself, so I pressed on. "Did you do IVF?"

If this emaciated woman, well into her forties, could conceive a child through in-vitro, then surely we could.

"No," she said, then averted her eyes.

Jamie rubbed my knee as the doctor opened our file and confirmed our health histories. I had expected her to sit us down and announce right away if we could have children or not. Instead, we had to answer a long series of questions. She started with me. I told her that I had hypothyroidism and pro-lactinoma. Before the prolactin medicine had regulated my periods, my cycles had been fifty-five to sixty days long. In my college years, I'd had two LEEP procedures to remove abnormal cells from my cervix. Otherwise, I was healthy. I told her that I exercised regularly, ate well. I was even starting to lose some of the weight I'd gained now that my prolactin and thyroid levels were normal.

The doctor moved on to Jamie who explained how his tes-ticular cancer had been misdiagnosed. He'd had a hydrocele—a sort of water blister—on his testicle at birth, and in his twenties, he'd noticed a similar thing. He went to his doctor, who took a look and said there was nothing to worry about. But it grew and grew until it became so uncomfortable that Jamie got a second opinion. His new doctor did a simple test, placing a light under Jamie's testicle. If it was a harmless hydrocele, light would shine through. If it was a tumor, it wouldn't.

Light did not shine through.

Jamie had a CAT scan and needed immediate surgery to remove the cancer.

He walked around thinking he was going to die. But after the surgery, his doctor said, "You're going to have a few months of chemo. It's going to be hell. But then you're going to have your life back."

At a time when all his friends were dating and partying, Jamie had to stop working and move home. He stayed on the couch in his parents' cold basement with the lights off and watched TV. His family drove him to the clinic, where he got his treatments through a port near his collarbone. The chemo made him nauseous, but Jamie and his mom joked that at least he'd get skinny for once in his life. Instead, Jamie bal-looned from all the liquids being pumped into him. He was swollen, pale, and bald. His friends hated seeing him this way, were afraid it would happen to them. They stopped coming around.

After Jamie was well again, his hair grew back curly. The first time Jamie was at a bar post-chemo, an old high school buddy came up to him and said, "Nice perm, dude."

Jamie simply said, "Thanks." He hated talking about his cancer, and was even more embarrassed to say "testicular." Now here he was, having to explain every last detail to a specialist we had just met. Sweat beaded on his forehead and his knee bounced an anxious beat.

The doctor nodded and scribbled notes, then, after a long list of questions about our family histories, she finally closed our file.

"You're great candidates for IVF," she said. She explained that because of Jamie's below-average motility and morphology, less invasive procedures—like the turkey baster method—weren't worth pursuing.

"But you'll have good odds with IVF," she said.

Jamie and I both exhaled. Our clenched hands relaxed.

She said that we had to time everything out, wait for the end of my next period. Then I'd begin taking birth control to shut down my natural cycle. I'd have to do daily injections, monitor my egg follicle development, and finally, when my body was ready for the egg retrieval, I'd go into the main office and have all of my eggs extracted. At that time, Jamie would give a semen sample. We'd go home, and the specialists would inject Jamie's sperm into my eggs. The fertilized eggs would grow in a petri dish. Three to five days later, I'd go back into the office and have the best embryos transferred into me.

I'll be pregnant in less than two months, I thought. It seemed relatively simple. I nodded and smiled, but Jamie searched my face with concerned eyes.

"Are you OK with this?" he asked. I could tell he felt bad

that all of the injections and procedures would be my respon-sibility.

I nodded and signed a stack of documents. I initialed *Yes* to the procedures. *Yes* to a pair of embryos being transferred. *Yes* to the paragraphs of fine print.

"I'm sensitive to everything," I cautioned the doctor as I signed. "I don't even like taking ibuprofen. So, I feel like we should be conservative with my doses."

"Of course," she said.

We could hear the lobby door open, and I knew that she had another appointment, so I asked one last question. "How about the side effects?"

She compared them to that of a period: mild headaches, moodiness. "Some women get hyperstimulation after the egg retrieval," she said, describing the condition of fluid imbalance, requiring hospitalization. "But that's rare," she said. "You're young and healthy. You're a great candidate."

Insurance must have thought I was a great candidate too, and they approved my cycle a couple weeks later. In fact, most women insured in Massachusetts got covered, which might just explain why I was seeing twin strollers everywhere.

The genetics workup was the only thing we were still waiting on. The blood test results would reveal if Jamie's and my DNA, when combined, might create a genetically troubled child. If so, then reproducing wouldn't be an option—naturally or scientifically.

But a week passed with no news. Finally, I called the lab, where a technician said, "Oops."

They had dropped Jamie's blood vial and hadn't called to tell us.

Jamie and I seethed and questioned if this was a sign of

trouble to come. But because we were so close to starting our cycle, we persevered, and Jamie got more blood drawn.

While we waited for the results, Jamie mentioned, almost casually, that if we conceived a boy, he worried about giving our son testicular cancer. Jamie was cooking dinner, and he stared at the stove the entire time he talked.

"Do you think it can pass down through my genes?" he asked.

I didn't know how to comfort him. Jamie rarely talked about the emotional impact of his cancer. But when he expressed his worries that our son might have to face the possibility of dying at twenty-four, like Jamie had, I could see the pain in his stare. I hugged him hard and didn't let go. The asparagus started to burn, and Jamie grabbed the tongs to flip the stems. Our conversation dissipated along with the smoke.

When I got my period, it was—for the first time in nine months—a desired milestone, because it meant the start of our IVF cycle.

Our genetic tests came back just in time. All was clear. The results felt like an advantage we had over other couples: we had irrefutable proof that our child would be healthy.

At Starbucks, over Labor Day weekend, as I prepped my lessons for my fall semester, I smiled at every woman who walked in with a baby. *Soon,* I thought, *that will be me.* I was due to start taking my birth control in a couple days, then I'd do the injections. I'd have my egg retrieval and embryo transfer sometime in early October. As I logged assignment dates on my course outline, I thought about how pregnant I'd be during each one.

Finally, I pushed my syllabi to the side and Googled "due date calculator." Noticing the other coffee drinkers at the nearby tables, I dimmed my screen and leaned closer to my laptop. When I typed in an estimated date for our embryo transfer, July 4 appeared in the due date column.

An Independence Day baby, I thought. *How perfect.*

As celebration, I went to an outdoor table and journaled. The sun warmed my shoulders, and I scribbled about the wonder of it all, how lucky I was—that I'd be pregnant in just over a month, that our baby would arrive after my academic year ended, that I'd get to spend all of July and August caring for our child before returning to teach at the university in September.

This time, next year, I thought, *we'll have a two-month-old.*

Oh, the good fortune of it all.

I wondered why more people didn't try IVF. It seemed so easy. Rather than trying month after month, charting ovulation, crossing fingers, crying with each period, couples could simply decide which month they wanted to get pregnant and control the entire process.

Chapter 6

The box arrived on my twenty-eighth birthday.

At first, I thought it was a birthday present from Dana. Then I saw "Village F Pharmacy" on the sender label and realized it was my supply of IVF medications. Jamie carried it from our porch to our dining room and set it on the floor next to a couple of presents he'd gotten for me.

Jamie handed me a birthday bag and I fished through the tissue paper to find extra-large elastic-waisted pajama pants.

"For future use," Jamie said, smiling. He talked about how cute I'd look with a big pregnant belly, and I forced a smile. Now that IVF was as real as the pharmacy box on our floor, I wasn't nearly as confident in my ability to get through the whole thing. For starters, the birth control pills I had taken for the last couple days made me unbearably nauseous. The nurses said the tablets were used to control my hormone levels and essentially shut down my cycle, but the only thing they were shutting down was my appetite. On top of that, my blood work appointment had made me thirty minutes late for class that morning. So, between my tardiness and constant puking preoccupation, I knew I was not setting a good example for my new students.

After blowing out my candles, I pushed my slice of chocolate cake around on my plate.

"Still nauseous?" Jamie asked.

I nodded.

"What did the doctor say?" he asked.

"Well, apparently, the only way to curb the nausea is to *insert* the pills."

"Insert them?" Jamie asked. "Where?"

I pointed down toward my lap.

"Seriously?" Jamie asked.

"Seriously," I said.

Jamie laughed, and I did too, despite my bad mood. Then the large box crept into my periphery, and I grew quiet.

Last week, a fellow English instructor had confided in me about her many failed cycles, how IVF had been so traumatic that she and her husband had opted for adoption. When I'd told my closest Massachusetts friend, Kelly, about IVF, I'd expected her to congratulate me. Instead, she nodded, carefully crafting her response. She had a coworker who had undergone two ineffective cycles. Sensing my disappointment, she said, "But that's not everyone's experience." Apparently it was. I had begun reading "What to expect with IVF" books, and I'd stumbled upon a vast field of troubling information. All of the women complained about painful injections, miscarriages. One stat I'd read kept haunting me: the average couple goes through three IVF cycles before having success.

I wasn't ready for any of it. I wanted a symptom-free, successful cycle. Was I gullible for previously believing that everything would be easy? What made us so special that we assumed we could just sign on the dotted line and get a baby?

Not wanting to alarm Jamie, I kept my apprehensions to myself.

He ate his cake happily and said, "You should really try a bite."

He had gotten the cake from a special bakery because I loved their chocolate ganache, so I forced a forkful, but it churned my stomach. How different this birthday was from my first one in Massachusetts, when Jamie and Tessa had donned birthday hats.

"I'm sorry," I said and stepped over the pharmacy box to get to the kitchen.

At the sink, I soaped up the sponge and looked out the open window at the tall trees that lined our backyard. A yellow tinge had painted the tips of the leaves and a few had even fallen. The temperature had dropped, noting the impending arrival of fall, and a breeze blew in, fluttering the pages of our calendar. It showed that I was due to start my injections in just a few days.

My arms goose-bumped, and I shut the window. Stepping over the box, Jamie joined me in the kitchen as I scrubbed our plates.

"So, are you going to open it?" he asked.

I looked at him, then at the box, and sighed.

"Alright," I said. "Let's do this."

Jamie carried it into the living room and set it on our large ottoman. I sat down in my leather chair, Jamie in his, and we looked at the big box that sat in the middle of us. We waited. Our lantern lights emitted a soft glow over the living room, giving me a momentary hopeful thought. Maybe it wouldn't be that bad. Maybe the women in my IVF books were just over-dramatic. Jamie handed me his keys so I could cut through the packing tape.

I wasn't quite sure what my overly optimistic brain ex-pected—maybe I thought that balloons or butterflies or fully formed babies would pop out and surprise us. Instead, I re-moved the bubble wrap to find stacked white boxes with long drug names like *leuprolide acetate—microdose leuprolide dilution.*

Then, printed underneath the names were numbers and measurements that frazzled my brain: *14 mg/2.0 ml, 75 IU.*

Every drug had fine print running vertically and horizontally around the package so that if I really wanted to read it, I would have to take out a magnifying glass and keep rotating the box. And forget the informational materials inside, with their pages of even-finer print.

Under the boxes were more white boxes containing two Gonal-f injection pens and interchangeable needle heads. Next to that was a tube of Crinone cream with a vaginal insertion applicator. When I dug deeper, there were yet more white boxes—larger ones containing alcohol swabs and gauze pads. Then I saw alarming reds—red-capped vials with liquid and powder, long needles with red covers, a large red sharps container. It was the size of a small shoebox, and I wondered if I'd really use enough needles to fill it. Like the medication boxes, it was labeled with fine print and foreign symbols, most notably, a large hazardous stamp. And the lid, which I couldn't open, was apparently adult-proof.

At the bottom of the box, there were leaflets breaking everything down into "easy" steps, but nothing was straightforward. Everything provoked questions. *Which medicines should I inject first? Where should I inject them? What time of day is best for injections? How large is my dose? Which size needle should I use? How the fuck am I supposed to open this sharps container?*

And the acronyms made my head spin. Every day, for fourteen days, I needed to inject a GnRH—gonadotropin-releasing hormone—and, then, nine or so days into that, I needed to start injecting an FSH—follicle-stimulating hormone. Then, before my egg retrieval, I would need to inject an HCG—human chorionic gonadotropin—trigger shot. After the egg retrieval, I'd start inserting the Crinone cream.

Since my "calendar" was regulated by my menstrual cycle, day five of taking Lupron might be day twenty-five of my menstrual cycle. This was somewhat straightforward, but once I started overlapping medications, forget about it. Day fourteen of Lupron was day six of Gonal-f and day three of blood and ultrasound work. How was I going to keep it all straight?

The pharmacy's tagline was written on the promotional materials, and I read it aloud: "Making fertility easier."

"Right," Jamie said, rolling his eyes.

What if I just repacked everything and set it back out on our porch for UPS to pick up?

I felt the way I had as a freshman nutrition major at the University of Illinois. The idea of it was great—my job would be to help others become healthy and happy. And then I had to take chemistry.

At my first class, I sat on the stairs of the overcrowded lecture hall with two hundred other freshmen. While they all scribbled away, I wrote not a single word in my notebook. The professor was speaking German. At least that's what it sounded like to my right-brained self. My mind worked in stories and emotional undercurrents, not numbers and formulas.

Now, the IVF booklet in my hand boasted similarly confusing calculations as well as websites with how-to videos. I pulled out my laptop and set it on the ottoman so Jamie and I could view the videos together.

The first video showed two hands and a vial against a black backdrop. I tried hard to pay attention, but there were too many steps.

I watched again and paused every five seconds or so.

"If the solution has air bubbles, get them out," she said.

How? I wondered.

"Inject in the upper outer thigh."

What exactly constitutes the upper outer thigh of a 5'2" female?

"Insert the needle."

How deep?

"Hold the needle in for ten seconds."

Approximately or exactly?

The second video left me baffled. It said to inject myself using a "dart-like" motion and rotate injection spots from my upper thigh, to my lower abdomen, to my triceps. I looked at the displayed diagram of a female body and almost laughed. *How the hell am I supposed to inject myself on the back of my own arms if Jamie isn't around?*

The videos were deemed supplemental to the meeting I should have already had with a nurse to go over such things in person—"should have" being the optimal term. In the IVF stories I'd read, all the women stated that they'd had a live demonstration as well as chats with the clinic's counselor to advise them on the stress they'd likely face.

I'd had neither.

Rubbing my temples, I picked up a needle package, then gulped at the length of the sharp metal.

"This is ridiculous," I said. "I need a nurse to tell me how this all works."

"You should call them tomorrow," Jamie said.

"By the way," he added, trying to cheer me up. "Greg invited us to go out on his boat next weekend."

I set the needles down and looked at him, wide-eyed. "Are you serious?" I asked, aware that I was being overly sensitive.

"What?" Jamie asked.

"You don't get it."

"What?" he pressed.

"This is going to be my life for the next month," I said, motioning toward the pile. "I don't think doing injections on a rocky boat is the best idea."

Jamie stopped talking and looked down at his lap.

It suddenly infuriated me—all the things I had to do while he had simply to fill a cup with sperm. But I buried it because I didn't want him to feel bad. I placed everything back in the box and continued on with the rest of our evening in a neutral mood.

We cleaned up the kitchen and watched a movie, and I said nothing about my fears or anger. At ten o'clock, I kissed Jamie goodnight and headed upstairs. When I reached the third step, Jamie called after me.

"I'm sorry that I have shitty sperm," he said.

Chapter

7

On my first injection evening, after viewing the how-to clip for the millionth time, I readied my dose. Jamie watched as I measured my medicine and cleaned my thigh with an alcohol swab. I sucked in a breath and hovered the needle over my leg. Then I exhaled and plunged it into my skin, pressing the syringe down.

After, I wiped the bead of blood with a gauze pad.

Looking a little pale, Jamie asked me how it was.

"Not as bad as I thought," I said. It was true, the injection wasn't as painful as I'd expected, but I still worried I'd miscalculated the dose or stabbed myself in the wrong spot.

"I don't know if I'd be able to do it," Jamie said.

I smiled and straightened up a bit. It made me feel good that he was proud of me. I felt proud of me, too. So, as I dropped the needle in the sharps container, I tried hard to discard my doubts.

As the weeks passed, the IVF preparation process consumed my life.

As soon as I woke up and packed my schoolbag, I headed for the blood lab. Because the clinic headquarters were so far from our house, I was allowed to go to a nearby hospital to have all my testing done.

At six forty-five, the waiting room to the blood lab would be full of elderly men socializing over Dixie cups of water as if sipping brewskies at the Elks Lodge. I'd frantically check the time on my cell phone while I waited for my name to be called.

This morning was no different. I waited a half an hour to hear "Johnstone," then the phlebotomist prodded the crook of my arm for a good vein. But instead of getting into my car and heading to work after I filled the blood vials, today I had to go upstairs for my first ovary ultrasound.

Though I could see what the injections were doing to my outsides—evident by the tender bruises that bloomed around my belly button and thighs—I couldn't see what they were doing to my insides, and that was the most important thing. This test would show if the medicine was working. And if it wasn't, that meant there was something wrong with the doses or with me. I'd have to stop this cycle and start all over again next month. *If* insurance approved, that is. Or it could mean that IVF wasn't right for us, and, well, I couldn't think about that.

When the technician led me to a small ultrasound room, I expected to lie on a table and pull up my shirt. Instead, she gave me a johnny and a sheet, and told me to undress. Then she left the room. I hadn't shaved my legs or my bikini line, and I felt embarrassed. The tech had obviously seen the effects of hormone injections before, but I was overly aware of my welts and bloated belly. I'd never been conscious of my ovaries before, but it felt as if they'd tripled in size. I'd barely been able to button my pants this morning, so taking them off now actually felt good.

The tile was cold on my bare feet, and I climbed onto the

table, the paper crinkling beneath me. A small computer screen blinked my last name. Near the desk, pictures of a girl in a softball uniform hung from a bulletin board, and I wondered if, soon, I'd be able to display pictures of our child at my work.

The tech knocked and came back in.

She pulled out a plastic rod that was a foot long, and covered it with a condom and lube, then said that it was time to insert it.

"Insert it?" I asked.

"They didn't tell you?"

I'd been asked this question the first time I'd gone to this hospital for blood work. "They didn't tell you which building to go to?" and "They didn't tell you that you needed to register first?" Today it was: "They didn't tell you that you needed an *internal* ultrasound?"

I shook my head. No—*they* hadn't told me anything.

The technician informed me that we needed to vaginally insert the ultrasound wand so she could view my ovaries. My injections were hopefully stimulating the production of multiple eggs so that the clinic would have many to fertilize at once. Right now we had to look at my egg follicles to see how many I had and how big they were. The tech also had to measure my uterus lining to ensure that it was thickening. But we couldn't see anything if we didn't insert the wand.

I swallowed as it slid in.

The tech used her left hand to type a few codes into the computer, and the ultrasound screen showed grayness at first. Then, as she maneuvered the rod, an oval appeared: my right ovary. Inside that oval were little chambers, like that of a honeycomb. These, I learned, were follicles that would produce eggs.

She counted over twenty-five follicles forming in my ovaries.

I felt like Frankenstein. Wasn't this a bit excessive? Did I really need that many eggs? Also, I knew that if my injection doses were too high, and my hormones became imbalanced, it could lead to hyperstimulation after the egg retrieval, which the specialist had mentioned. Though she hadn't given it much attention, I'd read that some women had to be rushed to the ER due to the nausea and dehydration. Liters of fluid needed to be drained from their abdomens. In this non-welcoming womb, the embryos wouldn't implant, or they wouldn't be transferred at all and all the injections would be a waste.

When I asked the tech if my follicle count was bad or good, she said that it was just her job to count and measure. My nurse would call me later with my results.

That afternoon, while I was meeting with a student during office hours, a nurse left a voicemail with numbers pertaining to my FSH, my estradiol, my follicle count, and my follicle measurements. I had no idea what any of it meant. When I called back, I got the nurse's voicemail. When she called back, I was teaching, and she left a voicemail to call her back. When we finally got a hold of each other on my drive home, she said, simply, that the medicine was working and that I should continue my injections and monitoring. She explained that everything was conditional, that the egg retrieval and the embryo transfer were never a guarantee. Each blood workup and ultrasound had to prove that I was progressing. The cycle could be stopped at any time if my hormone levels were off or if my follicles stopped producing.

My life became one long wait. I had never experienced such a thing. My teaching and writing blurred into the background, and the only thing in focus was the waiting. I waited at the blood lab, waited for my ultrasound, waited for the tech to count my follicles, waited for the nurse to call in the afternoon with my results, waited until eight o'clock to do my scheduled injection. I couldn't give the rest of my life much attention. My freshmen seemed too needy, their papers too daunting to grade. One of my favorite ESL students approached me after class and told me I didn't seem well. And forget faculty meetings. I was a body in the room that sat down and got up when other people did.

As Jamie and I spooned in bed one night, I explained how consuming the process was, how I wanted to press pause on teaching and press fast-forward on IVF so that I could get through it, get pregnant, and go back to my old life.

There were other things that I wanted to say, too, but they would only make Jamie feel bad. I wanted to say, *"I wish there were more things that partners could do and that IVF were a joint venture. I wish we could split up the responsibilities so that I'm only half as hormonal and half as preoccupied at work."*

He couldn't do any of these things, so there was no use uttering them. But there was one thing that was in his control, so, reluctantly, I said, "Can I ask you a favor?"

When he said sure, I rubbed his hand and asked if he could stay home from his work conference. He was scheduled to attend it in mid-October, which would likely fall on the same week as our egg retrieval. He was going to give his semen sample on the morning of the retrieval, and then fly out to his conference that afternoon. Jamie's mother would drive me home from the clinic and help me recover. But the more I thought about it now, the more I knew I needed Jamie's emotional support. I usually prided myself on my independence, but I needed him to come to the retrieval with me.

Jamie paused, then said he'd break the news to his boss tomorrow. I knew that Jamie was hesitant to cancel because he was new at his company and this trip would be a good opportunity for him to prove himself, and I felt a twinge of guilt, but some deep assertive voice shushed my worries.

"Jamie needs to be with you," the voice said, and it had such strong conviction that I believed it.

Over the next week, I tried to use this same confidence in becoming more of an IVF expert. By trial and error, I became more fluent in the lingo and the processes. I knew how to get the air bubbles out of my syringe, which route to the hospital lab was the quickest during morning traffic.

I grew to learn which of the phlebotomists were the best. The tan one with the neck tattoo always got my good vein in one painless attempt. But sometimes I'd get the older nurse with the cotton-ball hair. She'd scold my small arms or claim that I hadn't drunk enough water. My veins fought her jabs and pricks by collapsing.

Finally, one day, when the older nurse called me into the blood lab, I went up to the receptionist and requested the good phlebotomist. It felt so odd to be making demands, but my assertive voice spoke to me, asking why I was going to let someone mutilate my arms. Still, I felt bad about the awkwardness when the older nurse frowned at me as I passed her on my way to the tanned one's station.

Just like the phlebotomists, the ultrasound technicians also varied in personality and bedside manner. Each appointment meant a different tech, and each one would come up with different follicle or uterus-lining measurements. One technician gently maneuvered the wand toward my cervix and talked in a soothing voice, while another pushed it around inside of me so forcefully, I gasped.

This was the case with today's technician, who shoved the wand inside of me so deeply that I felt violated and had to dab my eyes with the back of my hand. As she pressed the long wand too hard and too far, I lay there, squirming silently. I didn't want her to feel bad, so I looked away, not wanting her to see my tears.

I hadn't come here to go down regret lane, but the persistent pressure of that wand inside me instantly triggered memories of the other times I'd lain flat while pretending that everything was OK.

The face that formed immediately in my brain was Nate's, appearing as arrogant as the day we'd met a decade earlier.

I'd started seeing Nate the summer I graduated high school. He was a college sophomore home on break and had a girlfriend in another state. His parents were always on vacation, so we spent most of July on his deck, listening to Dave Matthews and making out. During the day, I was a teacher's aide at a summer camp for kids with mental disabilities. At night, I donned halter-tops and too much makeup, trying to be the seductive woman that Nate desired. I wore a gold sequin top and platform heels the night I decided to lose my virginity to him. We hung out at his house and got drunk on his back deck, as usual. But afterward, instead of going home, I stumbled up to his bedroom and let him have all of me.

From then on, I fulfilled whatever fantasies he had, no matter how humiliating or degrading. I wanted so badly to see that look of satisfaction on his face, to please him. I'd always been that way. I'd gotten good grades to make Mom smile, won meets to make my track coach cheer. And I'd felt pride in each of these situations as others bragged about my accomplishments. With Nate, my pride came with the illusion that he preferred me over his girlfriend. But I found that I had to get drunker and drunker each time I slept with him. We never went on dates, and when I went over to his house, we no longer went to the back deck to listen to music. Instead, he led me right upstairs. And I followed him.

The last time we were intimate, Nate came to my house

when my parents were at work. I sat at our picnic table with a bottle of tequila that grew hot in the sun, and I downed three shots once I got word that he was coming over. He had to do a "deal" in my neighborhood, so my house was on his way, he said. He'd revealed this coke-selling job to me at the end of our summer fling, and, like everything else, I pretended to be cool with it. When he walked through the gate to my backyard, he—the coke dealer—raised his eyebrows at the tequila bottle.

"At eleven in the morning?" he said, but it didn't stop him from going inside with me.

In late August, he went back to his frat house and his girl-friend, and I went off to the University of Illinois.

I did plenty of things with guys in college, but I only went all-the-way with the couple of boyfriends I had. I was proud of the fact that I was regaining some self-worth, but I wasn't proud of the times I blacked out, unsure of the previous night's events—like the time over summer break that I woke up in a Vegas hotel room surrounded by passed-out guys I'd met the night before. I looked down, relieved that I was clothed. As I took a cab to my friends' hotel room, I hung my head out of the open window. My anxiety about what could have happened nauseated me, and I had to get belligerently drunk to drown the feeling.

During grad school, I continued to party and look for love, but I allowed myself fewer blackouts and fewer forays. One night, when I went back to a guy's place and told him I just wanted to kiss and talk, he couldn't get me out of his apartment fast enough.

"You could have at least given me head," he yelled.

So, it was no small relief to me that my first time with Jamie was the opposite of all these experiences. We had bonded during our three months of phone talking after meeting in Tampa. Each night, I'd chomp on my usual snack of Cinnamon

Toast Crunch and wait for my phone to ring, eager to hear about Jamie's day and tell him about mine. During my first trip to Boston, when Jamie embraced me at the airport with such warmth, I knew I'd be making love to him that night. After going out in the city, we came back to our room, each of us wanting to initiate something. Neither of us moved. Finally, Jamie reached into his overnight bag and pulled out a baggie full of Cinnamon Toast Crunch.

"So you can have your bedtime snack," he said, half-joking.

I grinned, then placed the baggie on the table, turned off the light, and took off my clothes.

Jamie moved in me with pure tenderness, reminding me that I deserved to be loved, respected.

But here, in the ultrasound room, there was no tenderness. There was only the technician shoving the wand around with no concern for my comfort.

I took a deep breath, gathering my courage, and said, "Can you go a little lighter please?"

"Sorry," she said, and the pressure released. I unclenched my leg muscles and exhaled, finding relief.

Though I could ask technicians how to maneuver the wand, I couldn't control how long it took for her to measure my follicles.

One tech might take five minutes to do the screening, while another took thirty, leaving me with no choice but to speed down the Mass Pike afterward, late, yet again, for class.

I used to hop around the campus from one class to another, but these days, I stood in front of my students tired and nauseous. My bloated belly threatened to pop the button off my pants. I ducked out of office hours and into hallways swarming with hungover nineteen-year-olds so that I could have hushed conversations with the nurses.

There were so many things about IVF that our specialist hadn't told us. She certainly hadn't described the track marks that would line my aching arms. She hadn't discussed how crazy I might become while on the hormones. These emotional shifts were nothing like the PMS mood swings she'd compared them to. One day, when I was showering and Jamie asked me to turn on the dehumidifying fan so that our bathroom paint wouldn't peel, I lost it. As soon as he closed the door, I growled, "Fuck you and your fucking fan," then cried under the water for the next hour.

Our specialist definitely hadn't told us how navigating through life while undergoing IVF was like having an affair. Because we didn't want to get our hopes up, or anyone else's, we didn't tell a soul. This meant a lot of lying. I lied to the women in my workout classes who asked why I had so many needle marks on my arms.

"They think I'm a heroin addict," I told Jamie after I came home from the gym one night.

"Right," he said, laughing. "All those heroin addicts that do boot camp classes."

I lied to my students about why I was always late. We lied to our friends about why we had to step out of the room when my phone rang with a call from the fertility clinic. I even lied to Dana. She was the one person, besides Jamie, in whom I could fully confide. I'd told her a bit about IVF, but I couldn't confess how overwhelming the process was or how alone I felt. If I complained too much, I worried that the universe might punish me with a failed cycle.

There was just one person I didn't have to lie to.

Mom.

I still wasn't talking to her, so I didn't have to worry about fabricating anything. But at night, when I did my injections, I secretly yearned for her pep talks. I needed assurance that I was doing everything right, and though she'd made me angry on countless occasions throughout my lifetime, she'd also encouraged me toward many of my accomplishments.

I thought about the day, during grad school, when I was moving into my studio apartment. Mom came to me with an envelope of savings bonds she'd been collecting since my birth—back when she was a broke nineteen-year-old in a troubled marriage, back when she had nothing but she wanted me to have everything. It was a few hundred dollars. "For emergencies," she said. And when I tried to thank her, she acted as if it was no big deal.

But when I considered calling her now, I thought about our fight on Mother's Day last year when she cursed me out for waiting until mid-afternoon to call her.

"If you were half the daughter I was . . ." she'd yelled.

Part of my subconscious defended myself. I was a good daughter. There were plenty of daughters that wouldn't put up with a minute of her drama. But then the other part of my brain thought maybe Mom was right. I had been a bad daughter. I'd been a brat as a child, a rebel as a teen. I'd been too self-involved in college and too stubborn to tell her I missed her when I'd moved to Massachusetts.

And if she was right, that I had been a bad daughter, then what kind of mother would that make me?

Chapter

8

Feeling upset that IVF had taken over my life, I planned to steal back some of my former freedom and independence. I joined a weekly writing class at a writing center in Boston. Grub Street was, for me, the Columbia College of the East Coast. When I'd moved to Massachusetts and missed my grad school community from back home, I did a Google search for writing organizations in Boston and discovered Grub. For every term since then, I'd been taking and teaching creative writing classes there, and I was determined that this fall would be no different.

Each trip to Grub Street was a treat. I drove into Boston with the same excitement as when I used to take the train into Chicago. Tonight was no different. I smiled even as I inched along the congested traffic. It filled my soul and my writing muse to see the throngs of people in Copley Square buying sunflowers and mini pumpkins from the farmer's market.

After I parked, I stopped at Starbucks for a latte and walked toward the Steinway Piano sign—the landmark building that stood next to Grub Street. So much about this past month had felt foreign, but this certainly felt like me—coffee, writing, the city. Yet, as I wrestled my heavy laptop bag up my shoulder while trying not to spill my drink, there was something that most certainly felt "not me"—the large lunch cooler hanging off of my right arm. My scheduled injection was at 8:00 p.m., and this class lasted from six thirty to nine thirty, meaning that I'd have to do my injections in Grub Street's tiny bathroom.

I'd signed up for the class to work on my novel, but during tonight's in-class writing time, I drafted a letter to our future child instead. During our mid-class break, a group of students headed down the narrow hallway to wait for one of the two bathrooms, and I followed, toting my lunch cooler and uttering a silent plea, *Don't let anyone stand in line behind me.* It'd be so much easier if I could just hang a sign on the knob that said "Injection in progress," and warn everyone that it would be a while.

Tonight's HCG trigger shot would take even longer than usual. It was the one we'd been waiting for, the one that prepared my ovaries for my egg retrieval—which we'd just found out would be on Tuesday. I had to mix a specific amount of powder with a specific amount of diluent. It meant two different measurements, two different vials, and two different needles.

In the bathroom, I opened the cooler and surveyed the inventory—alcohol swabs, vials, needles, sharps container. This bathroom wasn't as dirty as the burrito joint bathroom I'd had to do my injections in the other night, but this was certainly more cramped, and I could barely move without bumping into the toilet and the sink. My notebook contained the steps I'd scribbled while watching the how-to video, and I pulled it out now.

1. Place the long needle into the diluent. 2. Draw back 1cc of air with the long needle. 3. Inject the air into the vial, then pull back 1cc of diluent. 4. Plunge the contents into the vial of

powder. 5. Shake it until the powder dissolves into liquid. 6. Change needles. 7. Pull back the entire contents of the powder/diluent mixture. 8. Grab belly skin. 9. Inject entire dose.

I took a deep breath and forced my shaky hands to follow each step. Outside the bathroom, people talked and laughed, alerting me that other students were still waiting in line. The door to the adjacent bathroom opened and closed twice while I did my preparations and people were definitely wondering what the heck was going on in my bathroom. Then, just as I hovered the needle over my stomach, someone knocked on the door. It startled me so much that the needle almost flew out of my hand and into the toilet. This would have ruined everything. It would have wasted the only HCG powder I had and forced me to miss the specific injection time needed for egg retrieval preparation.

Somehow, I held on to the syringe and caught my breath.

"One second," I yelled at the door. Then I jabbed the needle into my belly.

Emerging from the bathroom with my lunch cooler, I lowered my eyes and scurried back to the classroom. But when I sat down, relief accompanied my exhale. The hard part was over. All I had to do now was go to my egg retrieval on Tuesday and have my eggs taken out and fertilized in a petri dish. I'd be back to work on Wednesday and Thursday. On Friday or over the weekend, my fertilized embryos would be transferred into my uterus, and I'd return to work with a baby in my womb.

My life would be barely interrupted.

During this class next week, I'd be pregnant.

Chapter

9

What do you do when you know your life is about to *change?*

I pondered this question on our drive to the fertility clinic for our egg retrieval.

How could I function when I was going to be pregnant in just a few days? How could I sit in Jamie's passenger seat, admiring the fall leaves and listening to Ray LaMontagne on the radio? How could I focus my attention on anything else besides the baby that would soon be growing in my belly?

I wasn't thinking about the retrieval as a procedure to extract my eggs or even thinking of my eggs as eggs. I was thinking of them as miniature MEs that would soon be combined with miniature Jamies, which would then be planted into my womb. And, there, one perfect little being would bloom.

At the clinic, we climbed the stairs to the second level where a set of doors separated us from our future. Jamie smiled at me and we sucked in a deep breath, then reached for each other's hand. When we stepped into the patient prep area, I half-expected to see a ward of pregnant women or a nursery full of newborns—something to indicate that this was the place where babies were made, where babies were guaranteed. Instead, the nurses gathered at a station in the middle of the floor, which was encircled by curtained sections. Though the space was less exciting than I'd anticipated, the windows flooded the patients' beds with sunlight and the air smelled much less antiseptic than the hospital where I usually got my blood drawn, a promising sign.

After initialing a stack of consent forms, I put on a johnny and a pair of booties. It was a bright October day, but my thin gown made me cold, and my chilly limbs were grateful for the heated blankets the nurse offered me. While we waited for our names to be called, Jamie and I sat in our little unit with the curtains open, as did the other patients. It was like we were all tenants sitting on our balconies, facing the same courtyard. Even though we pretended not to, we were all studying each other. An Indian couple occupied the space to our left, the man older than the woman. Had his issues brought them here? The woman to our right lay on the bed in a post-procedure haze alone, and I wondered what her story was. Was she a single woman trying to get pregnant on her own, or was her partner on a business trip like Jamie would have been if I hadn't asked him to stay? One thing was certain: Infertility affected people from all walks of life, regardless of gender, race, or age. It surprised me that the other women here were around my age. Each of them appeared to be younger than thirty.

Finally, a nurse alerted us that it was time for me to head to the retrieval room.

Sometimes, I wished I could capture Jamie's expressions, like the sideways smile he had right then when he leaned down to kiss me before the nurse led me away. It was his most adoring look, and his eyes crinkled with love. His gratitude filled his gaze—that I had made it through all the injections, that we were so close to creating our child. I smiled back, as a way of thanking him for missing his business conference to be with me.

The nurse brought me into a dark room with equipment and a large screen, which would magnify and project my ovaries. Since our doctor was booked with appointments today, I'd be in the care of the two doctors who stood on either side of me in scrubs.

They explained the process—how they'd sedate me, then go through my cervix to extract all of my eggs with a thin syringe.

I leaned back on the examining table, shaking with nerves and excitement while the female doctor instructed me to bend my knees and scoot forward. One minute, I was putting my feet in stirrups, the next minute I was out.

When I awoke, I was back in our curtained-off section with Jamie by my side. He grinned at me and smoothed my hair behind my ears.

"Hi, Monkey," he said.

Feeling like I had just woken up from a nap, I looked around to get my bearings. My lower abdomen, which I'd expected to be sore, felt fine. My nurse smiled and said that the doctor would come talk to us in a minute. The papers in her hand listed all of the potential side effects of the procedure, and she pointed at them as she explained the most severe complication—hyperstimulation, known as OHSS. It was the thing I'd been dreading ever since the specialist had mentioned it during our first appointment. The nurse explained that sometimes the ovaries become swollen and painful, throwing off the body's hormonal balance and compromising the fluid levels. "You might throw up or have diarrhea," she added. She left out the part I'd read in the books about an ER trip to drain excess abdomen fluid.

The nurse recommended a low-carb diet and plenty of liquids to help reduce fluid retention. We'd already purchased things like Greek yogurt and coconut water, which awaited me at home. I asked her if I had to stay in bed for the day, but she shook her head and suggested to just take it easy. She added that in the unlikely event I had to call the nurse hotline, the number was listed on the bottom of the handout.

I hoped we'd never have to look at it.

Jamie carefully folded the papers and slid them into his pocket. Then the female doctor who had performed my retrieval came by to tell us that they had gotten a good amount of eggs.

Jamie rubbed my arm. This was the best outcome we could have hoped for. More eggs meant higher odds of having two well-developed embryos to implant into my uterus. And two embryos meant higher odds that one would survive and thrive.

The doctor nodded about the good news, but there was something lurking in her expression, and she glanced at us warily before walking away.

"Alright," our nurse said, as she patted the foot of my bed. "You're free to go."

I glanced at the clock over her shoulder, shocked at how early it still was.

"That's it?" I asked.

"That's it."

As Jamie and I drove away from the fertility clinic, we kissed and held hands.

"We're going to have a baby," I chanted as we drove.

A baby. A baby. A baby.

Due to our fear of jinxing, we'd only recently disclosed a few of the details to Jamie's parents and my sister. Now, Jamie called his mom and dad. He smiled the entire time he spoke. Jamie was usually so neutral in expression that he was hard to gauge. His face maintained the same appearance no matter if he was elated or enraged. He absorbed everything, but rarely reacted and was the only person I knew who stood completely still at rock concerts. There was one time I'd seen him break his neutrality—when I'd surprised him with a two-night stay at a luxury lodge on Moosehead Lake in Maine. When we walked into our room, he didn't jump up and down the way I would have. Instead, he called his parents and bragged about every last detail of our suite—the lake view, the furniture made out of birch wood. And he was like that now, boasting to his mom about how well I'd done, how many eggs the doctors had extracted.

I scrolled through the names in my phone, wanting to dial every relative and friend to proclaim that we were just days away from being pregnant. But I wasn't sure if my Chicago friends would quite understand my strong desire for a child, or the lengths I'd gone to. In their late twenties, most of my girlfriends were still single or dating. The ones who were married weren't thinking about kids yet. Just weeks ago, when I'd told Courtney that Jamie and I wanted a baby, she'd said, "A baby? As in a small human?" Then she'd asked, "Don't you want to do more before you have kids?" I was both furious with her reaction and relieved that I hadn't confided in her about IVF. Last week, I'd sent her an email stating how hurt her judgments had made me. I couldn't accept that her concerns might carry some weight, that my other friends probably felt the same way. Though Jenny would be much gentler in her tone, I knew she might ask, "What's the rush?" the way she had three years ago when I announced I was moving to Massachusetts for Jamie.

I also wondered how Mom would react. My thumb hovered over her name for a moment, and then I put my phone in my purse so that I wouldn't be tempted. Our months of not talking had been cleansing. My life felt so much less dramatic without her in the picture. She'd never seen our new house, knew nothing about our daily life. So, it felt like Massachusetts and our home were sacred and untainted. And with us not talking, I no longer had to worry about saying something that would upset her, nor did I have to worry about Mom saying something that would upset me. There was some truth in the notion that it was healthy to cut toxic people from your life, even if they were related to you.

Still, it was lonely.

"I feel like I don't have a family," I'd told Jamie just last week. Besides Dana, I wasn't in contact with most of my Chicago relatives. And the more time I spent with Jamie's polite parents, the more embarrassed I became of my dysfunctional uncles and cousins.

"We'll make our own family," Jamie had said. But I wasn't sure if starting fresh in Massachusetts and cutting off Chicago was completely healthy either. My move had certainly helped me discover who I was without outside influence. But wasn't it also cathartic to accept and embrace your roots?

It was too much to think about right now. I didn't want to ruin this happy moment with worry. So, I decided that Jamie and I should do something fun together with our day off.

When we stopped at the Alcott's Orchard House, I seemed fine at first. I moved normally and even felt upbeat. Then, halfway through the tour, my legs wished for a chair. Standing required too much energy, and I leaned on Jamie while the guide took us through the upstairs bedrooms. My dizzy head and hot skin were reminiscent of a hangover. Thirst left my tongue dry, and I knew I needed to drink something so that I wouldn't get dehydrated.

By the end of the tour, I was desperate to slump into the passenger seat of Jamie's truck and close my eyes. I reclined the seat, then inclined it again, then reclined it once more but couldn't get comfortable. Jamie stopped at a convenience store, and I chugged half a bottle of a red Gatorade, then felt queasy.

Once home, I crawled into bed, determined to rest, and Jamie went to the local diner to get us breakfast. I had to lie on my stomach so that the counterpressure of the mattress could help alleviate the soreness of the cramps that seized my entire abdomen. My stomach churned and ached, making me feel full and nauseous all at once. In my tired brain, a nagging thought persisted, questioning if I was hyperstimulated, but for some strange reason, my shoulders also hurt horribly, as if knives were lodged into them.

By the time Jamie returned with our food, I was a mess. He tried to get me to eat, but I took two bites of my omelet and had the immediate urge to vomit, so he helped me down the stairs, guiding my wobbly limbs. Once in the bathroom, I grabbed the toilet seat to steady myself while I threw up red liquid that I hoped was Gatorade.

Jamie suggested calling the doctor, but I didn't want to be a wimp. He held his cell phone, ready to dial, while I tried, between bouts of vomiting, to dissuade him. The nurses had said my abdomen might be uncomfortable, and I didn't want to overreact or be humiliated by going to the ER unnecessarily. But I couldn't stop the searing pain in my shoulders or the corset of spikes spearing my stomach.

After stumbling to the living room, I collapsed on the couch and buried my head in my hands, releasing a different sort of sob than I had ever uttered. It didn't come from anger or overt emotion. It was as if my subconscious knew what was happening internally and wanted to expel the suffering. If I wouldn't admit that some serious chaos toiled within, my tears would express the message for me, and it was signal enough for Jamie.

"I'm calling," he said and dialed the nurse hotline. He listed my symptoms, and if I had been on the phone, I wouldn't have even mentioned my shoulder pain because that didn't seem IVF-related, but when Jamie communicated this, the nurse ordered us to the ER.

"You might have internal bleeding," Jamie said after he hung up. For my benefit, he hid any trace of worry. What would be happening right now if Jamie had left on his business trip and his parents were taking care of me? Would I be silently suffering in their guest bedroom, afraid I was overreacting, only to fall into a sleep from which I'd never wake up?

Jamie led me to the back door as he gathered keys and insurance cards. In my compromised state, the seriousness of the situation didn't register. I actually felt relieved that the diagnosis wasn't hyperstimulation. I still hadn't considered the cause of my bleeding or how the doctors would correct it. There was an episode I'd seen once on the show *ER* where a man and woman were impaled by a metal pole, and the doctors hesitated removing it because this would trigger the internal bleeding to worsen, which would kill them both. This was the only reference I had for "internal bleeding" and I ranked my situation as far less life-threatening than that.

I'll be fine, I thought.

But fine I was not. As Jamie grabbed our sweaters, I stood in the doorway to the porch and wavered. The room shifted, and bile climbed up my throat, so I staggered to the bathroom to throw up once more. Again the liquid was red. When the nausea let up for a moment, Jamie told me to lean on him so he could slip on my shoes. Then, unsteady as I was, I couldn't step out of the house on my own, so Jamie picked me up and carried me through the door.

During our five years together, he had carried me for plenty of other reasons—like when I'd embraced him at the airport during our long distance days and refused to unlock myself from him, and he'd shuffle us to his car, laughing all the while. He'd carried me through our front door when we'd purchased our house. But he'd never carried me because I was physically unable to carry myself.

When he strapped me into the passenger side, the pressure of the seat belt seized me and I shrieked. I reclined the seat, trying to get comfortable, but the farther down the backrest went, the less I could breathe, the more it felt like I was sinking into the mud of my own body.

Every bump in the road during the fifteen-minute ride made me clench my stomach and moan.

The hospital was the same one I'd gone to for all of my blood work and ultrasounds. It seemed like a bad omen that I was going to the same place where the older phlebotomist had cursed and stabbed me, where the oblivious ultrasound tech had pushed the wand around inside of me without any concern for my comfort. *Is the rest of the medical staff as careless?* I wondered.

The nurses rushed me through the lobby—past every sick, groaning person—and into a curtained-off area. Though it was similar to the fertility clinic's prep area I'd been in just hours earlier, here the chaos of the beeping machines and patients' shouts made everything more urgent.

The assertive thoughts that I usually censored found their way to my mouth now, requesting antinausea meds and insisting that my bed be kept at an angle because lying flat made me feel as if I were drowning. In a sense, this was true. My own blood was saturating my lungs.

A young doctor came in to perform an ultrasound of my abdomen to locate the source of my bleeding. In order to do this, I needed to lie flat as he pressed a probe to my stomach. Despite my pleas to keep the bed at an incline, he insisted that he could not, and when he reclined the bed, I gasped for breath. My hands groped the air to be pulled up. Couldn't the nurses see that I was suffocating? Why would no one save me? Worried faces circled my bed, but they couldn't do anything to help me.

The doctor pushed the wand down on my lower abdomen, and I yelped. The pain was unbearable, but I had no choice other than to cry and let him continue. He and the nurses theorized that maybe my uterus had been nicked or lacerated during the egg retrieval. Still, I didn't anticipate how the doctors would fix this.

Either from the loss of blood or the pain, my brain fogged, my focus waned. Jamie had to do most of the talking. An OB surgeon—a tall old man in scrubs—came in and said that the ultrasound had revealed a mass of blood, no telling where it was coming from and no time for laparoscopy. I needed surgery, and I needed it now.

I sat on the bed moaning, looking around in a daze, not realizing that "surgery" meant he was about to slice me open. Jamie's cheeks blazed. His eyes searched mine. For the first time since I'd known him, his calm composure disappeared.

"So what happens now?" he asked, panic filling his voice. The surgeon replied that they weren't sure what they would find, and he needed Jamie's permission to perform a hysterectomy on me if necessary.

This made me howl in such a primal way that I didn't even recognize my own voice.

"I'm only twenty-eight," I sobbed. "I've never had kids."

The surgeon responded that he would have to do what he would have to do.

"My highest priority is saving your life," he said.

So Jamie nodded and held my hand as I wailed. Then, without warning, the nurses and doctors rushed my gurney down an endless white hallway to the OR prep room. Jamie ran alongside it, looking like he might faint, while I gripped the metal bars and pulled at my IV, begging someone to tell me what would happen to our embryos. Would we still get to implant them in three days? But the surgeon's crinkled face above mine didn't answer my questions. Instead, he gave orders to the other doctors in a medical language I couldn't translate. It didn't matter. I had no control over what was about to happen to me.

In the small room full of wires and beeping monitors, the medical staff hurried around me, securing a mask over my mouth. Jamie's face hovered over a doctor's shoulder in the doorway. They told him he couldn't accompany us to the OR and that he had to go to the waiting room.

I counted backward as Jamie mouthed, "I love you."

Then he waved goodbye.

PART II

Chapter

10

When my eyes blink open, I see a bulging stomach covered by a hospital gown and legs with compression cuffs that inflate and deflate. I see an arm with a port for pain meds. I see a body that I realize, in horror, is my own. Machines beep and a monitor displays my vitals, and when I try to sit up, my middle feels like it has been sawed in half.

"Hi, sweetie," Jamie says, and I find him sitting to my left with bloodshot eyes and uncombed hair. My arms reach out to hug him, but my core fights back, warning against any twisting, so he leans over the bed bars and holds me gently, like he's afraid to hurt me. His eyes tear up as he kisses my face and intertwines his fingers with mine.

"That was so fucking scary," he says, shaking his head. "I thought I was going to lose you."

At first, I'm not sure what he's talking about. *What was scary?* I want to ask. I don't know what happened or how long I've been asleep. My memory is blank. The only clue is that the hospital room is sunny, which means I must have slept here after surgery. Surgery. Flashes of memory start to fill my mind. The ER. The doctor saying I needed surgery. But everything after that is foggy.

"What happened?" I ask Jamie. He's wearing the same red shirt and carpenter jeans as he did yesterday, but now they're creased in odd places from a night of sleeping in the recliner.

"It was your left ovary," he says. "It never clotted after the retrieval. But everything's fine now."

My lungs release a long exhale, but then I remember the obstetrician asking Jamie for permission to do a hysterectomy.

Is that why my abdomen hurts so badly? Did they have to re-move everything?

Panic flushes my cheeks. *What will I do if they removed my uterus? What will happen to me if I can't be a mother?* I pull at my johnny to look for evidence of a hysterectomy, but I can't even lean forward on my own, my core feels so sore. Panic quickly escalates me into hysterics. The room tunnels. My hands grab at my gown. If I learn that the doctors took away my chance to be a mother, I'll lose it.

Jamie places his hand on my arm. "What's wrong, Nader?"

In a desperate voice, I ask, "Did they have to . . . ?"

Jamie looks confused.

"Remove everything?" I finish.

Please say no, please say no, please say no.

Jamie shakes his head.

I take a deep, thankful breath that fills my whole body.

"Oh thank god," I whisper, almost reverently.

Jamie tells me how, last night, he paced the waiting room for two hours, thinking about how he was going to lose me and how he'd have to call my family and tell them I had died. Every time the door opened to the waiting room, he jumped and his heart stopped. Then, finally, the surgeon came in and gave him a thumbs-up.

"I hugged him," Jamie says, "and then I collapsed into a chair."

"What about the embryos?" I ask. "Can we still implant them?"

Jamie glances at my stomach, and I can see he's trying to find the right words.

"The doctor said we can try in about six weeks, but you need to recover first."

"Recover from what?" I want to ask, but by the way Jamie keeps looking at my abdomen and handling me so delicately, I know last night's surgery must have been more invasive than I thought it would be. *How did they access my ovary?* I wonder. *What kind of cut did they have to make?*

Before I can investigate what's going on beneath my hospital gown, Jamie reaches for my hand. "You should leave it alone. The doctor says that it's healing really well."

We sit in silence for a moment when it occurs to me that I should probably be at work right now.

"What day is it?" I ask. Jamie says Wednesday, and I realize that I'm scheduled to teach in an hour. Right now I should be driving to the university while mentally prepping my lesson. Tonight I'm supposed to grade papers and answer emails and write a chapter for my Grub Street class. But I imagine that the doctor won't discharge me until this afternoon, so I won't be doing any of these things. For someone who prides herself on checking off a long to-do list, this realization does not sit well.

I've never canceled class last-minute, and I reluctantly dial the university's number. When the department secretary answers my call, I have no idea how to explain my situation.

"I'll be back tomorrow," I tell her and Jamie tries to signal me, but I hang up.

"I think you'll be here for a few days," he says.

"A few days?" My brain feels heavy, confused. My eyes droop.

Jamie pats my arm and says I should get some rest.

"What are you going to do while I sleep?" I ask.

"I'll just be right here," he says.

Love isn't proven by wedding rings or vows. Proof of love is in the way that Jamie takes care of me. When I wake up from my nap, Jamie is waiting with a cup of water and a straw. He anticipates my needs even before I can utter them. As I sip my water and lie on the bed, he presents me with crackers and gossip magazines. He strokes my hair and encourages me to press the button for medication at regular intervals so that the pain doesn't get ahead of me.

The surgeon knocks on the door and smiles at me. I remember his wrinkled face from yesterday, but it's strange to see him standing there calmly, not rushing my gurney down a hallway. He says that after he made the incision and found my left ovary, it looked like Swiss cheese from all the extraction needle pricks. He had to take the ovary out of my body and hold it in his hand to compress it before he sutured it.

"You're one lucky lady," he says.

But when Jamie leaves to go home and let Tessa out, I don't feel lucky. I feel lonely. A nurse knocks on the door, saying that she has to change my dressing. *What does she mean?* This hospital speak is strange to me. Not since having tubes in my ears at the age of two have I been admitted to the hospital. I've never sprained an ankle or broken a bone.

The nurse lifts my gown, revealing my stretchy hospital underwear.

How big is the incision? I want to know. *How bad does it look?*

When she pulls down my underwear, I see a long strip of gauze running from my belly button all the way down to my pubic bone. The length of it makes me nauseous, and I have to look away. If I look down, it will be real, and my heart can only handle so much right now. The nurse wipes my skin and applies a new bandage, but all the nerves in my abdomen are numb. I feel the pressure of her fingers and nothing else.

Vanity seizes me. *I'm only twenty-eight*, I think, *and my body is already ruined.* I think of Mom, of her ruined body, of her C-section scar. The first time I ever saw it, I gagged. It looked like a shark had bitten her. The pink, jagged line ran from one hip to the other.

"A botched job," Mom would explain later. "That's what happens when you give birth at a military hospital." And she was right. It was botched. Although Mom had a toned, flat stomach, the muscles in her lower abdomen never fused back together correctly, and the scar tissue made her flesh zigzagged along the incision.

My first memory of it was when Mom was getting out of our bathtub. She was drying off with a towel she had confiscated from a Best Western. Behind her, duct tape secured a garbage bag over the crumbling shower tiles that we couldn't afford to fix. I was standing on a small blue chair, brushing my teeth. The sight of her stomach made me choke on my toothpaste. She wrapped the towel around her small body, sat on the closed toilet lid, and lit a cigarette. The towel split open at her waist, and there it was again, the scar.

When I was growing up, and we'd get into fights, Mom always told me that I wouldn't understand her until I had kids. And though our bodies were so alike, it seemed that her C-section scar was the major divide between us. Because I wasn't a mother yet, she reasoned, I couldn't possibly know what it was like to be one. It was true, I didn't know what it was like to sacrifice so many things, even the perfection of the body, for someone else.

But based on the size of the gauze pad, my vertical incision is even bigger than her horizontal one. Now that my body feels like damaged goods, I'm realizing everything my incision represents—loss of independence, loss of optimism. I'm starting to feel like I might just have an inkling of the things Mom has been through.

In her last voicemail, Mom said she'd give me my space, honor my decision to not talk anymore. It felt like a relief when I heard those words. I thought, *Finally, she's thinking about what's best for me instead of herself.* But now, I crave her. In my youth, on my rare sick days, Mom set me up on the couch with a TV tray of oyster crackers. She flattened a bottle of Sprite and poured it into a yellow cup. We watched *Beauty and the Beast*, which was my favorite Disney movie, then *The Little Mermaid*, which was hers. She was always so busy folding clothes and washing dishes that it was a gift to have her there with me, just sitting, just being my mother.

But as a teenager, I felt self-sufficient and got confused when Mom tried to discipline me like a parent. When I fell in love with Jamie and Mom got upset with me for moving, I wanted her to view me as an adult capable of making my own choices. But now, I want her to be my mother again. I want Sprite and oyster crackers. I want *Beauty and the Beast* and *The Little Mermaid.*

I want to be her daughter.

In the hospital hallway, a family passes, carrying balloons and flowers to another patient's room. I think about who will visit me. Though Jamie's parents live near us, they are at their lake house in Maine for the week. Mikey and Kelly are tending to Tessa after they get home from work so that Jamie can be here with me. All of my friends and family are in Chicago. I will have not a single visitor. No one even knows I'm here.

Strips of sunlight move around my hospital room as the afternoon passes. The dark creeps in, as do some troubling thoughts. I don't know if it's the nighttime or the alarming beeps of other patients' machines. Maybe it's the pain meds. Or maybe it's because I'm usually so busy that I've never sat with my thoughts before. It's like forced self-reflection, emotional rehab. Every single thought that I have ever buried resurfaces now.

At first the thoughts are those of longing:

I miss Chicago.

I miss my friends.

I miss my family.

Then they are self-pitying:

My body is ruined.

Why did this happen to me?

If I were in Chicago, this room would be full of visitors.

Then the thoughts turn to questions:

What if I'd been more patient and hadn't jumped into IVF?

Would this have happened if we hadn't gone on the Alcott tour?

If I were in Chicago, would I really have a room full of visitors?

What about the extended family I never talk to?

What about friends, like Courtney, that I've pushed away?

What about the sister I rarely contact?

What about the mother I've chosen to ignore?

I don't like sitting with these thoughts or facing their answers. My finger yearns to press the nurse call-button. To ask for what? Food? Painkillers? I know that there is nothing they can offer me that will take away the truth that I'm just starting to face.

On the nightstand, my phone dings with a text message, a welcome distraction. I try to lean forward to reach it, but it's two inches from my grasp. My labored breaths inhale air that reeks of sterile plastic and urine. My arms tangle in my IV tubes. My catheter tugs at my groin. My incision feels like it will burst open where my ab muscles are flexing.

Finally, panting, I reach my phone. It's a text from Jamie, telling me he's on his way back. It dings a minute later, and I assume it's him again, but it's a message from my friend, Marie, wishing me a smooth recovery. Next, Jenny texts, followed by Katy and Sarah.

Jamie must have told everyone. Then the phone makes a startling noise that sounds foreign. It's ringing, and a glance at the screen reveals that it's Mom.

Another shrill tone fills the hospital room, and I know there are three rings left before it goes to voicemail.

My thumb hovers over the button while my stubbornness challenges my vulnerability. As badly as I want to talk to her, is it healthy to do so while I'm feeling this desperate? What if I answer and she scolds me for not talking to her, for not telling her about IVF? I'd yell so loud my stitches would pop.

The phone rings again, forcing me to make a decision.

Just before it goes to voicemail, I answer.

"Nadine?" Mom asks, shocked, concerned.

I can't talk. My bottom lip quivers.

"Nadine?" she asks again.

"I'm here," I whisper.

"I can fly in and take care of you," she says right away.

As an answer, I start crying.

"I know," she repeats. "I know."

When I regain my breath and dry my eyes, I'm drunk on truth and I tell her about everything—wanting a baby, going through IVF.

She listens.

"I can fly in," she repeats, "if you want me to."

My thoughts teeter between begging her to get on a plane right now and insisting that I don't need any help. If she does

visit, I imagine the long afternoons of silence that would surround us, forcing us to talk about all of our anger and resentment. I'm not sure if I'm quite ready for it, or if it might make
my recovery worse.

"Thank you," I say. "But I'll be OK."

"Are you sure?" Mom says. "I can get on a plane tonight."

"I'm OK," I say.

"I love you," she says.

My heart wants to return the words, but my brain fights
them.

"Thank you for calling," I say.

We hang up, and I decide to confront something else before my brain talks me out of it.

I move my johnny and pull down the hospital underwear
to reveal my gauze-covered flesh, then peel away the medical
tape from my abdomen. As preparation for what I'm about to
see, I suck in a deep breath and strip back the cotton pad.

Look down, my brain says, and I do.

There's a harsh pink line, folds of flesh that were sewn
back together like the bunched-up stitching on badly hemmed
pants.

It's even worse than Mom's. It is so incredibly ugly.

The air in the room is so heavy that I have a hard time
breathing. There's no ignoring or fleeing from the reality of
my midsection. I have a large, jagged incision that will turn
into a large, jagged scar that will never go away.

A nurse doing rounds knocks on the door next to mine. I
scramble to replace my bandage, then pick up a gossip magazine and pretend to read.

When I flip it open, a body lotion advertisement stares
back at me.

A flawless midriff covers the entire page.

Chapter

11

My appetite is small and I feel full after eating just a fourth of my hospital breakfast, maybe because I am still so bloated and everything is pressing up. Maybe it's because the surgeon left some of the loose blood in me to be reabsorbed so that I wouldn't need a blood transfusion. I go through my morning routine of taking my iron pills and exhaling into my breathing machine, begging the plastic balls to reach the top of the tube. Because of my decreased red blood cells and lack of oxygen, when I breathe out, the balls struggle just to lift. It feels like trying to blow up a pool raft that has a hole in it.

"This thing is broken," I tell Jamie, handing it to him.

He barely breathes into it and the balls go right to the top, so he hands it back and tells me to keep practicing. Instead, I put it on my nightstand and tell the machine to fuck off.

I used to wish for a catheter. When I was comfy and warm in bed, and the urge to go couldn't be ignored, I'd throw back the blankets and joke about the device saving me from a trip to the downstairs bathroom. But now that there's a catheter wedged up my insides, I'll never wish for one again.

I have to pee but don't know how.

"Just push like you normally would," the nurse says. But there is no normal anymore. Jamie looks at me encouragingly, and I push but don't feel liquid moving through my body. When my desire to empty my bladder disappears, I assume I've gone.

The complete loss of independence is maddening. I can't sit up without inclining the hospital bed, can't move around without a wheelchair, can't stand up to take a shower. I can't even poop without stool softeners.

A nurse comes in to give me a sponge bath, and I cringe, mortified, as she helps me undress. My unsupported chest sags to either side of my body. My armpits sweat. My full catheter bag rests near my unshaved legs.

But the nurse doesn't stare. She doesn't complain. She runs the sponge along my arms gently and takes great care around my bandages. When the sponge travels between my legs, I look away and want to cry, but she cleans the area with such gentleness that I want to hug her and say thank you. Right now she is the mom and sister and friend that I don't have in Massachusetts.

Time has paused for me, but the rest of the world keeps moving. Two days here have felt like two years. My initial belief that I'd be discharged after twenty-four hours is laughable. After an exhausting series of x-rays and body scans, I'm wheeled back to my room, and the nurse suggests that I try to transfer my body from the chair to the bed. But how can a person move when their core muscles have been completely severed? Despite my determination, I need Jamie's arm for support. So, when the doctor says I'll be here another couple days and that it'll be another two weeks before I can drive or work again, I believe him.

The next day, the nurses move me to a shared unit, and my roommate is an elderly woman who has a long list of ailments. Our room tastes of disease and death. The staleness is dizzying. Smells of bleach and gravy mingle together. The air is too warm.

When my catheter is taken out, my trips to the bathroom become what I dread the most. I have to shimmy off of the bed and grip my IV stand for support. Standing up straight is not an option, lest I want my incision to rip open, so I hunch and shuffle to the bathroom. The twenty feet from my bed to the toilet take me about ten minutes to navigate. My roommate always leaves her lights off and watches the news in the dark, so my trips past the foot of her bed always disrupt her TV viewing. In the bathroom, I have to bend and put my urine sample basin into the toilet, then lift my johnny and squat down. With an abdomen that has been sliced in half, my core is not strong enough to support my upper torso, and my hand grips the handicap bar shakily.

I am afraid to pee because it burns as the little flecks of scab from inside my urethra tear off. Then I just want to stay on the toilet for the rest of the day, because pulling myself up is worse than sitting myself down. My left ovary feels like a ten-pound dumbbell tied to a thread that is yanking at my insides. With one hand on the handicap bar, I use my other hand to tug my underwear up. This alone takes a good five minutes, seeing as how my IV and my johnny keep getting in the way, but tying my gown shut is too much work. Since one hand always grips my IV pole for support, I have to wash my hands one at a time. *How is it possible for a hand to scrub itself?* I wonder. Hopefully hot water kills all the germs. By the time I shuffle back to my bed, it's nap time.

That night, our skinny infertility specialist comes to visit me, and I sense that she's questioning me to see if I'm likely to sue the clinic. When I ask her why this happened to me, she explains that these are the risks that I signed off on when I initialed my paperwork. I am part of the small percentage of patients who experience the things in the fine print.

"Maybe," she says, "the batch of needles we used for the retrieval were too sharp. We're looking into it."

Family and friends advise us to take the clinic to court. They use the words "fault" and "malpractice." They say, "with all of today's medical advancements . . ."

Jamie and I talk about what went wrong and theorize that the clinic wasn't conservative enough with my dosages, so I produced many more eggs than I should have. I was overstimulated and poked one too many times during the egg retrieval. But we'll never know if that stop we made to Louisa May Alcott's house forever changed our fate. And because we don't have the money to consult a lawyer and take on a huge organization that will surely have a ruthless legal team, we decide to just move on.

I can't reverse events. I bled internally. I went into surgery. I have a scar now. There's nothing we can do about any of it.

There's also nothing I can do about the approaching nighttime.

Jamie and I sit on the right side of my bed, facing out toward the window. I try to imagine that we're sitting on a park bench in the Boston Common watching the sun set over the swan boats. Jamie caresses my hand and kisses me. He tells me how much he loves me, how he was terrified of losing me. There's so much love looping around us.

But then, visiting hours end. Now that I'm in a shared room and in stable condition, the nurses say that Jamie has to go.

The dim hallway light filters in through the curtain as my hand clasps Jamie's, and I trace the Celtic knots on his wedding band—our symbol of unity, of bonded strength. I don't want him to leave me. If he stays in the chair and just passes out there, the nurses will look the other way. But Jamie needs to let Tess out, and he is a follower of rules, so he packs up to go.

Maybe Jamie needs a break. As hard as it is for me to be the one recovering, maybe it's even harder for him to be my sole caretaker. Maybe the moment he steps out the doors, he feels relieved. And who could blame him?

Tonight, though, I need him here for more than just company. I can feel the anxiety growing with the darkness in the sky. The nighttime is when my mind races. "An idle mind is the devil's workshop," Mom used to say. But tonight, it's more than that. A nagging worry speeds my pulse: What if, when I close my eyes, I never open them again?

The nurse enters to check my vitals, and Jamie fishes his keys out of his pocket. *How can I tell them the crazy thoughts in my head?*

"Can I have some anti-anxiety medicine?" I ask softly. Jamie stops zipping his coat and squints at me, confused. The nurse looks at Jamie.

I have an expired prescription for Lorazepam in our medicine cabinet that's still full because even though I've struggled with anxiety, I try to avoid medicine at all costs. But tonight I need a heavy dose of something.

"Why do you need medicine?" the nurse asks.

I don't want to say it, but if I don't, there might not be any relief from this persistent panic.

"I'm afraid I'm going to die."

Again, the nurse looks at Jamie, silently asking if this is normal.

Jamie sits down on the side of my bed. "What's wrong, Nader?" he asks.

The nurse checks the compression cuffs on my legs and asks why I think I'm going to die.

An image keeps flashing in my brain and won't leave—me in the OR prep room with doctors rushing around me. Jamie mouthing "I love you" and waving goodbye, me fearing that when I close my eyes, I'll never open them again.

I don't know how to explain this or if they'll even understand.

"I'm afraid I won't wake up," is all I say.

The nurse tells me to hold on a minute and leaves the room.

She comes back with a pill that I swallow in one sip.

Jamie holds my hand until my eyes grow heavy, until they finally close.

When Jamie comes the next afternoon, I show him my latest talent—walking—something that I took for granted just three days ago, back when a stroll down the hallway was something I did about fifty times a day at the university. Now, it takes us an eternity to make it to the elevators. We press the down arrow and it feels like we're escaping when we roam the lobby.

At the automatic doors that lead outside, I look over my shoulder, waiting for some hospital guard to wrangle me and order me back to my room. But the workers and doctors are all preoccupied with their own problems.

Outside it's cold, and, God, does it feel good. It's the freshest, crispest air I've ever inhaled. My johnny billows in the wind and my nipples skim the fabric, but I don't care because Jamie is holding my hand and helping me hobble down the sidewalk.

Cars whiz by us, on their way home from work, and I think about what I'd be doing right now if my ovary hadn't bled. *Probably leaving the university and heading to yoga*, I think, and then I pause. *No, today is three days after the retrieval. Today I'd be having my embryo transfer. Today I'd be carrying our children.*

"The clinic called," Jamie says as if reading my thoughts. The wind whips my hair and he brushes it out of my face.

"We have nine embryos," he says. "They're being frozen so we can use them later."

I imagine the embryos suspended in little blocks of ice, just waiting for me to heal so that they can be thawed and given life.

But how long will they have to wait for me?

The sun sets behind a building, and I shiver. The parking lot and street grow fuzzy with the darkening sky, and night closes in. Jamie suggests we go back inside, but all I want to do is climb into his truck so we can drive far away from this place.

An ambulance races to the hospital entrance, its sirens screaming of trouble, and my fears of dying encroach me. Even though I will be discharged tomorrow, even though my body will eventually heal, I wonder how long it will take for me to recover mentally. *What if I never do?*

Chapter

12

When Jamie brings me home the next afternoon, it's a relief at first. But because I can't traverse the steps, the couch is my bed. At 10:00 p.m., Jamie kisses me goodnight and heads upstairs as the dark living room closes in on me. There are no nurses or machines to monitor me, so I could die in my sleep and no one would know. Usually walking would help me calm down, but I can't make it more than two blocks without assistance, and I'm not about to shuffle through our neighborhood at midnight. So, it's just me and the dark night and my dark thoughts.

I wake up feeling like I'm drowning. Even though I dozed off while sitting up, my body must have shifted into a flat position. My lungs feel saturated, and I gasp for air as I search the room for Jamie.

The October sun shines brightly through our bay window and the clock reads 8:30. There's a note from Jamie on the ottoman saying that he didn't want to wake me so he left for work. I'm alone.

What if I'm bleeding internally again, and the blood is flooding my organs?

This panting isn't right and I need to see a doctor, but who can take me? Jamie's mom is back from Maine and is the only person I know in Massachusetts who can help me.

"Can you come over?" I ask, panting.

When we get into Judi's car, I punch the doctor's address into the GPS and lean back in the seat so I can rest while she drives, but when I open my eyes, we're stopped on a side road, which is backed up due to construction. It doesn't seem like we're headed the right way. Judi admits that she's not good with directions, and then I notice that the GPS has sent us to the wrong town. Worry floods my gut. *What if I can't breathe and we get stuck here, in the middle of nowhere?* The more I worry, the more rapid my breathing becomes, and in no time I'm in a gasping panic attack.

Judi keeps glancing at me, sweating, unsure of what to do or where to go. My anxiety feeds off of her frazzled expression. In turn, her frazzled expression feeds off of my anxiety. And so the frenzied cycle goes. We don't know where we are and why the GPS won't recognize the doctor's address.

I really don't want to call Jamie. It's his first day back to work, and surely he has a million things to deal with, but there's no one else in Massachusetts who can help me. So, Judi calls him. I want so badly to get out of the car, off of this back road, and in a vehicle that is headed to the doctor's office.

Jamie leaves work early and directs us to a gas station where he meets up with us. Ever the face of collectedness, he directs Judi back home and helps me into his truck.

At the doctor's office, I have a full sobbing meltdown in the crowded lobby. I'm crying because I feel bad that Jamie had to leave work early. I'm crying because the one day that he left me in someone else's care, I still needed to seek his help. I'm crying because there is no one else who can take care of me. I'm crying because I don't know what's going on inside of my body and why I can't breathe. I'm crying because I'm not pregnant, and I should be.

The receptionist calls me in to see the doctor, most likely because I'm disturbing the other waiting room patrons with my sobbing. The doctor looks at my incision, which he says is healing well, but I disagree. Each time I've cleaned it over the past twenty-four hours, I've been shocked to see how long and bumpy it looks. My left abdominal muscles bulge more than my right, proving that the cut was not symmetrical. To me, "healing well" would mean erasing the incision and getting my old torso back.

As for my labored breathing, he thinks that there's some loose blood left inside of me.

"It's still trying to get reabsorbed," he says. "I'm going to readmit you to the hospital just to make sure everything is fine internally."

After tests and scans at the hospital, the doctors confirm that I'm anemic and still reabsorbing the loose blood, so they keep me overnight for monitoring to ensure that I'm still stable tomorrow before they send me back home. After Jamie leaves, that night in the hospital is the worst night of all. I pace the room, shaking, thinking, *What if I lie down and stop breathing in my sleep and never wake up?*

My anxiety triggers unrelenting diarrhea and each push of my intestines threatens to split my incision. When there's nothing left to expel from my body, I lie in bed and call Jamie's cell for the security of his voice.

"I'm not going to die in my sleep, right?" I say.

"You're not going to die in your sleep, Nader," he says in a tired tone.

It's got to be exhausting for him—taking care of me and the house and the dog and work. Now he has to worry about his wife being a mental patient.

My finger hovers over Mom's name on my cell phone. How badly I want to dial her and Dana and my friends and say, "Please, come. Come as soon as you can."

When the nurses take my vitals, I talk to them at length so they'll keep me company. If they are watching over me, I believe that nothing bad will happen to me. When they leave, the TV keeps me awake until dawn peeks through the blinds, and I doze off.

The next day, after calling the university and asking for more time off, I hear a knock at the door. A middle-aged woman with wavy hair stands in the doorway.

"I'm a social worker here at the hospital," she says, then she sits down in the chair next to my bed and asks if I'd like to talk. She seems nurturing, and it's nice to have a visitor.

"My husband and I were doing IVF," I say, and I'm about to continue when she cuts me off.

"A lot of people struggle with infertility. It's more common than you think."

"Yeah," I say, "I'm learning that." But when I start back into my story, she interrupts me again.

"IVF can be really stressful," she says.

That's what I'm trying to tell you, I think, *if you'd just zip it and listen for a minute.*

But she doesn't listen. She talks and talks until tears reach my cheeks. She touches my arm, thinking it's a cathartic moment, but I shift to the right side of the bed, out of her grasp. Jamie and the doctor walk in just as I'm reaching for the tissue box on my tray.

The doctor sees my red eyes and asks what's wrong, but all I can do is shake my head and look away.

"Buck up," the doctor says. "You should feel fortunate that you have all your organs."

Anger rings in my eardrums and my lips tighten into a

line. My body hardens with rage and rotates away from him, as if shielding my fragile core and fragile soul. I think of Mom and the many times she threw plates around in the sink, screaming, "What about me?" My fury could break a whole set of china.

Jamie stares at me, wondering what I'm going to do.

When the doctor stops talking, I turn my head back toward him and stare at his crinkled face with burning eyes, as if possessed. My voice is a guttural growl.

"If one more person tells me that I should be grateful," I hiss, "I'm going to fucking lose it."

Then I do lose it—sobbing into the starched bedsheets, ignoring the doctor and the social worker until they leave.

Jamie rubs my back, and I feel, in his palm, how heavy of a responsibility I've become.

Even while crying, I make a decision to get my act together. I'm going to keep my hurt to myself, not burden Jamie or his mother or anyone else. When the doctors discharge me from the hospital again, I will take care of myself alone.

So that's what I do. Back home the next morning, Jamie gets ready for work, and I sit out on our cold sunporch with a book. Though every ounce of me screams, "Don't leave me!" I plant a smile on my face and wave goodbye to Jamie.

His face relaxes when he climbs into his truck, and I understand that this is how he copes. When he goes to work, he gets lost in emails and phone calls. The business of his job carries him away from our IVF trauma and my neediness. He gets to be Jamie Johnstone, operations manager, and not Jamie Johnstone, childless caretaker of a needy wife. Then, when he comes home, he escapes into television and food. He can watch Dave Chappelle and laugh or get caught up in an action flick and fantasize about life as a Navy Seal. He can snack at night and numb his emotions. Whereas I grapple with my stress outwardly, in the messiest way possible, Jamie uses distraction.

Judi says she can come over today and Mom repeats her offer to fly in, but I insist I'm OK.

Through trial and error, I learn which medications I should take and when—iron pills, stool softeners, ibuprofen. I learn that Percocets are not my friend. I learn how to take naps sitting up. I learn how to clean my incision, but I still haven't learned how to accept that it's there. Once the gauze is peeled back, I stare down at it for a long time, my fingers running along the cut, which is nauseatingly numb.

Anxiety is a new permanent state, and if I carry Lorazepam around, sometimes it gives the placebo effect without having to place the pill on my tongue. Still, the negative thoughts circle my cerebrum. It seems that when the doctors cut me open and held my hemorrhaging ovary outside of my body, they also exposed every repressed worry and every harsh truth I've ever stowed away.

My brain busies itself by watching the neighborhood, and during my first time at home on a weekday, it becomes quickly apparent that absolutely nothing happens here. The only person I see is the mailman who comes at ten.

Each day, I wait at the door for his deliveries—Jenny sends me a care package; my ESL students make me a get-well video; Marie, who unexpectedly lost her young mother in August, sends me a touching card about loss; Courtney, Mom, and Dana send flowers even though I've been nearly absent in their lives.

Dana and I make up for all of the talking we didn't do over the last four years. Although she is only twenty-two and just graduated college, she speaks like a therapist who's been counseling patients for decades. She says all the right things, like, "This must be so difficult. You're dealing with a lot right now. You have to take care of yourself."

When did she get so wise? I wonder. In the years I've been away, she's morphed into an amazingly empathetic person.

"Thank you, sister," I say before I hang up, but there's so much more I want to say.

Remember all those times in high school I screamed at you for wearing my clothes?

I'm sorry.

Remember when I visited you only twice in your entire four years at college?

I'm sorry.

Remember when your ex-boyfriend pushed you and I disregarded it as a drunk fight?

I'm sorry.

Remember when you confided your secrets to me, and I questioned you instead of consoling you?

I'm sorry.

And you know what some of my favorite memories are? When we'd camp in our little rental cabin in Michigan every summer. You and I would take our mattresses off of the bunk bed and put them together in the living room and we'd stay up late, talking side by side. I loved that.

You know what else always makes me smile? When we'd write messages on each other's backs with our fingers. We'd write silly things like butthead, *but then, every now and then, one of us would write* LUV YOU.

And each year, when Mom hid eggs on Easter, I loved running around the house with you to find them. You laughed and elbowed me out of the way. You always got more eggs than I did. You were always so determined.

And I felt so proud of you each time I watched you play soccer and each time I helped you get ready for your school dances.

I've never told you, but I was always so jealous of the easy way you made friends, and how you brought them in close to you. You weren't afraid for them to see all sides of you. You and your friends could laugh and fight and laugh again. I always cut people off as

soon as they said something I didn't want to hear or made even the
most minor mistakes.

I'm realizing now that when I moved to Massachusetts, I gave so much of myself to my new life, my new love, that there wasn't anything left for anyone else. Now, I'm seeing the repercussions.

During this extended time alone, recovering, I sit in our living room and think about all these things. In the afternoon, I linger in each room of our lovely home and feel such loneliness that it seizes me. We've put so much heart into this place—I picked out the serene green paint on the walls and the colorful pillows on the couches; Jamie has updated all of our floors and light fixtures. Every room is bursting with color and life, but then I step out onto the porch, and everything outside is dull and dormant. Even though we live near a main road, it leads to a laundromat and a Salvation Army. Three miles in the other direction is a pizza joint. I yearn to walk to a coffee shop just to sit and be around people my own age.

How did we move to a place so different from my Chicago apartment? What made me ignore my concerns about moving to a remote town two years ago, when we were looking for houses to buy? I'd felt increasingly more isolated the farther outside of Boston we searched, but each Saturday, we continued to tour homes that bordered farmland.

My memory pauses on the night shortly after we purchased our house. Jamie and I were walking Tessa through our small neighborhood, and I grew silent. The stillness of the street, the lack of people—it instantly depressed me.

Jamie asked what was wrong, and my eyes averted his gaze.

"Oh, I'm just happy," I lied.

"For now," he said, picking up on my tone.

I nagged him to elaborate, and finally he sighed, then cleared his throat.

"I just think you'll always want more. I don't think that this"—his arm waved out at the sprawling land in between each house, the goat farm in our neighbor's backyard—"I don't think that this will ever be enough for you."

We stood there, in the middle of the street, no noises coming from the houses, no neighbors getting into their cars. It was as if someone had pressed pause on life here. Jamie's words hung, stagnant, between us: "I don't think that this will ever be enough for you."

"It is," I insisted.

Because I wanted so badly for it to be.

Chapter

13

Two weeks after my surgery, I ease myself into my car for the first time and readjust the seat belt that cuts painfully across my incision. Worrisome questions fill my brain, like: *Will braking hard make my insides spill out of the slit in my middle?*

But now that my body is securely fastened in the driver's seat, the real question is, *Where should I go? What do I need in order to heal from this unexpected trauma?*

I need healthy food and new clothes, I need Tuesday and Thursday evenings at Starbucks to write, I need games of Bananagrams with Kelly, I need laughter with my ESL students.

But the thing I need most is yoga.

My bloated stomach still protrudes; my incision still tingles with pain. I haven't consulted any doctors to ask if I can exercise again, because, quite frankly, I don't trust them anymore. After what has happened to me, I've concluded that *my* mind, not a doctor's, is the one most in tune with my body. And my mind tells me that what I need right now is church, or at least my form of worship, which is yoga. It seems as if every yuppie has turned to yoga for some quick conversion to Buddhism or merely to show off their cute capris, and I can't say that I haven't bought into the hype, but for me, especially today, it's not about any of that.

Wisps of lavender and cardamom tickle my nose when I enter the quiet studio.

Linda, the owner, stands at the counter, wearing her usual bandanna over her short hair, and I've come to her class today because she gives the most personal attention of any instructor I've ever had.

"I can't do all the poses," I say. "I had surgery on my abdomen . . ."

How do I phrase this? I wonder. *What kind of lie can I make up?*

Then my wiser mind asks, *Why do you need to lie? Is it because, god forbid, your surgery involved a reproductive organ? Why is an ovary something to be ashamed of? If you had broken your foot, would you lie about that?*

"I had some complications," I confess, "after an IVF procedure."

I expect Linda to ask what IVF is or to recoil, as if I am a mad scientist doing cloning experiments in my basement. But Linda nods knowingly and hints that she, too, went through reproductive assistance before having her daughter. The bell on the door rings, and another yogi approaches the counter, so Linda gives me the *If you ever need to talk, I'm here* look. I have yet to join an infertility support group or an online forum, but talking to her feels like a start.

The heated studio almost instantaneously draws sweat from my pores, which is another reason why I am here: to move, to test my muscles, to feel Linda's healing touch, but, really, to sweat. I can feel the drugs and the negative energy and the anger pushing at the surface of my skin, urging me to open the valve and release.

Skinny women in Lululemon stretch on their fancy mats. If any of them see the bulge of my bloated abdomen under my baggy clothes and ask if I'm pregnant, I'll run out of the studio. Though I'd usually stand front and center, I don't want them to wonder why I can't participate in most of the poses, so I place my mat in the back left corner of the studio instead. Spreading out the purple rubber, with its little flecks missing from years of hand and footprints, is like coming home.

Like the girl to my right who looks to be in her late twenties, I used to wear formfitting tank tops. I used to do crow and headstand. Now, I'll be able to do maybe an eighth of the poses.

Do I belong here anymore?

I feel infinitely older than three weeks ago when I last stood on my mat. My soul feels ancient—not in the mature sense, not in the wiser sense, but in the sense that life has hardened me.

When Linda comes in, we begin in child's pose and the surrender makes me want to weep and smile all at once, clear evidence of my emotional instability. In mountain pose, I stand tall, proud, but I can't stretch fully or arch backward for fear that my incision will burst open. I am so much more careful than I've ever been, going through the poses slowly, learning this new body of mine. What can it do? What should I push it to do? What must I avoid?

My limbs go right from forward fold to downward dog. I don't have the abdominal strength yet for high push-up or low push-up, and I certainly can't put pressure on my core in cobra. With the pulling and tugging and twisting, most of the postures are inaccessible to me.

But I can do tree and chair, and for these things I am grateful.

I sweat like I haven't sweated in so long. It feels so damn good. I can feel it pouring out of me—the IV fluids, the stool softeners, the iron pills, the ibuprofen, the Percocet. I can actually feel the detoxification. But the best part is the assists—someone else guiding me. When Linda gently repositions my arms, it feels so incredible to be helped, to be supported.

What a gift touch is, one I still don't know how to receive. During shavasana, final resting pose, Linda puts her hands between the mat and my upper back and pulls, gently encouraging my neck to lengthen, my spine to expand. The cardamom oil on her fingertips soothes my mood. At the base of my head, she cradles my skull and massages my tense neck muscles. Then she slides her fingers over my ears and smoothes my temples and forehead. Sweat makes my skin slippery. Hair escapes from my bun in untamed tufts. My mascara smudges my eyelids. My foundation streaks down my face.

Still Linda rubs.

Because I haven't received any form of motherly touch in years, I don't know what to do with my gushing gratitude. I've starved myself of nurturing female contact for so long, that I am just now discovering the gaunt cheekbones and protruding ribs that must be my psyche. I yearn for Mom to reassure me, for Dana to hug me, for a friend to pat my forearm. *Why oh why did I ever believe that I didn't need them when I moved to Massachusetts?* I ask myself. *Why have I been so careless with their love?*

After class, endorphins and relaxation move through me, lifting me ever so slightly out of the muck of my mind. Though I am far from healed or from forgiving myself, I feel a half inch closer. When I peel off the layers of my damp clothes, I am shedding layers of negativity.

Thus begins my thrice-weekly practice. Every time I go, my need for warmth and touch is met. On cold November afternoons when it is already dark at four-thirty, I enter the studio smelling the lavender and cardamom. Then I kneel down on my mat, and I am healed.

I'm doing well for weeks, and my body reflects this. Thanks to my yoga practice and a strict diet, my weight drops and my muscles tighten. Surprisingly, my abdominal fibers fuse back together and the swelling subsides. Still, my dark scar runs, jaggedly, down my middle and my left ab muscles bulge more than my right. Luckily, our bathroom mirror at home is not full-length so I don't have to catch a glimpse of my carved stomach every time I get out of the shower. When changing after yoga class, I'm always sure to remove my clothes in such a way as to hide my stomach. No one besides Jamie has seen my scar, and it feels like a secret. There's no outward proof of what I've been through, so I don't have to talk about it, and yet I want to wear a pin that says, *Tread cautiously, I've been through some shit recently.*

I'm fitting into clothes I wore a year ago, before all of my hypothyroid issues came to light, so my health kick is enough to distract me from obsessing over my childless state at all hours of the day. I'm even finding joy in teaching again, especially now that I can get to class on time and stay focused. But when we get the bill for embryo storage, it goes immediately into the shredder after I pay it. Although I could do the transfer soon, I'm just not ready yet. But I can't explain why.

Mom and I talk once a week or so now. It's awkward sometimes. We're so used to screaming and holding grudges that talking honestly and respectfully feels like navigating new territory. My heart is hungry to draw her in but also afraid of being hurt.

Mom says that the period of us not talking taught her a lot of lessons. Though she rarely apologized during my youth, now she says sorry repeatedly—for being overbearing, for being unsupportive of my move.

I have a policy—anytime I think about censoring myself with her, I don't. She has to know my honest feelings. So, I admit that those things did hurt me. A lot. Instead of being defensive, as she normally would, Mom listens. In turn, I tell her all the things I regret—what a brat I was as a teenager, how, when I moved to Massachusetts, I was too stubborn to admit that I missed her.

Little by little, I begin to mend the rifts I've made with everyone I left behind in Chicago, but I still have a lot of work to do. Each time I call Dana, I ask about her life and try to talk about mine less. I want to be as involved as I can be, even if it's just over the phone. I email and text my friends, and I realize that I didn't call Marie nearly as often as I should have when she lost her mom. If my IVF trauma has made me feel alone, surely she feels ten times lonelier. I dial her number more often now, if nothing but to listen.

And then the holidays approach.

I want to embody the peaceful spirit that I do in yoga class, but bitterness and jealousy encroach along with the winter wind. Anytime I see a mother holding her child, an angry envy consumes me unlike anything I've ever known.

There are public areas I must avoid now—the kids' section at Target, the corral of cribs at Ikea. I can't even read gossip magazines that headline pregnant celebrities. Our Vitello bib remains hidden in my dresser.

Then there are the triggers that I can't possibly predict.

On Thanksgiving, I am not thankful. In fact, as we plate our turkey and sweet potatoes, I'm counting my misgivings: my six-inch scar, my heightened fear of dying for no particular reason, and, the worst misfortune of all—my barren belly.

We eat dinner sitting around Jamie's cousin's living room.

Making small talk, I pretend to be the same upbeat person I was the last time we gathered here, even though I will never again have the obliviously optimistic mind-set I did a year ago. After we clear our plates, I sip wine and try, unsuccessfully, to convince myself that having shiraz and a slimmer stomach is better than having a child.

I baked Grandma Kenney's Irish bread to trick myself into thinking that I'm at Thanksgiving in Chicago, but it's not working. Dana calls, and I take my phone into the bathroom with me. She has to yell over our rowdy relatives playing Left Right Center and clanking beer bottles behind her. When she asks how things are in Massachusetts, I lie and say I'm having a fantastic time, but when we hang up, I sit in the bathroom for ten minutes avoiding the politeness and civility that awaits me. As cordial as Jamie's family is, they could be the image of perfection, and still, they wouldn't be my Chicago family.

Wasn't this one of the benefits of coming to Massachusetts—to cleanse myself of my shit-faced, shit-talking relatives? So what's possessing my desire to hop on a plane and sip Jager alongside them?

It was my decision to leave them, I think. If I go crawling back, it will be as if I'm saying that moving to Massachusetts was a mistake, that none of this would have happened if I had stayed in Chicago.

Family. The word vibrates in my wine-buzzed brain.

When we all leave Jamie's cousin's house, it's a relief that I won't have to pretend to be happy for the next half hour as we drive to Jamie's Nana's for Thanksgiving-number-two.

But then, out on the dark driveway, as we're about to get in our car, Jamie's brother, Josh, lights up a cigarette, and his wife, Ciara, says that, due to her newly heightened sense of smell, even a whiff of smoke repulses her.

We stand there on the gravel drive for a second, all of us

with hands on car door handles, ready to get into our different vehicles. The night is so black that it's hard to make out people's expressions, but Jamie's mom keeps fidgeting with her purse, looking back and forth between Josh and Ciara, like she knows of the announcement they're about to make.

"I'm pregnant," Ciara says.

And just when I think I'll collapse right there, Ciara tells us that the baby is due the first week of July, just as ours would have been.

Chapter

14

Maybe I'm just oversensitive. Maybe people are just overly ignorant. Maybe it's both. But, lately, it feels like everyone's saying the wrong things to me.

Everyone tells me to just relax. They ask me if I've considered adoption. They proclaim that everything happens for a reason. But if they even think about asking me if we're going to try transferring our embryos soon, it will tip me over the fine edge of hysteria on which I'm always teetering.

When Jamie and I visit his mom one Sunday, she opens the door grinning, exuberant. Judi says she has something exciting to show us and waves us to the study, where her computer screen displays an ultrasound of a family friend's baby. She exclaims over the skinny limbs and tiny toes.

Jamie sees the angry hives crawling up my neck, the narrowing of my eyes. He squeezes my hand.

How could she? I think.

Then she leads us to her kitchen, and her refrigerator displays more ultrasounds, but of a different baby. It's Josh and Ciara's baby, Judi's first grandchild—the grandchild that Jamie and I had hoped to give her.

Unbelievable, I think. *Is she messing with us right now?*

If I were in a more rational state, I might reason that she has every right to brag about these babies. I mean, why should she have to hide her happiness?

But I'm not rational. And I'm not taking the high road. I'm definitely not being the better person. No, no. Instead, I wince in my woundedness, and I cut our visit short without explanation.

Days later, I call Judi to tell her how hurt I was during our visit. As comfort, she says that she knows people who have tried for almost a year before they conceived. But this is not at all reassuring to me. In fact, it's another reason I'm convinced that no one understands me.

"Trying to conceive naturally for a year is very different from not having the option at all," I say before hanging up.

It's bubbling up—the need to do something extreme. Things that used to console me are no longer effective. Wine nights with Kelly help a little and yoga takes off the edge, yet the anger still stirs in me. Usually, I'd write about it, but I can't bring myself to type a single word. At home, I look out the window at the snow, and a word repeats in my brain: *Escape.*

If I were a drinker, I'd go on a binge. If I were a slut, I'd have an affair. If I were a rebel, I'd get a tattoo. But what I am is a fleer, so I'm going to travel somewhere far, and I'm going to do it alone.

It's been my coping mechanism for my whole life. At seventeen, I went off to college and rarely visited home on the weekends. After my freshman year, I moved in with my much older boyfriend for the summer to avoid Mom's dictatorship. The day after I was handed my master's degree, I moved to Massachusetts for Jamie.

Whenever I'm feeling off, I leave the house. I go for jogs,

drive to coffee shops. The heavier the emotion, the farther I go. Last year, to escape my winter blues, I went alone to El Salvador and taught there for two weeks.

So, now, with the crushing weight of my jealousy and anger, I know a simple trip down the Cape isn't going to cut it. I need to get out of the country.

On a frigid winter's day, I receive an email from my friends and fellow Grub Street instructors, Jenn and Adam, inviting me to a writing retreat in Guatemala. Adam had sent the initial email in the fall, but I'd disregarded it as impossible. Now, it calls to me. The pictures show a writing hut on a glistening lake surrounded by volcanoes. Vitamin D and story workshops are exactly the medicine I need right now. I don't *want* to go to Guatemala. I feel, with absolute certainty, that I *need* to go there, that I *must*.

I don't consult Jamie. I don't want his practicality. I don't want the guilt. Instead, I write an email to friends and family announcing my plans and I cc Jamie on it. It's a coward move so that I don't have to squirm through a face-to-face conversation and lay out all the reasons why this trip is a necessity, not a luxury. Plus, even though the money we earn individually should be considered "ours" in a marriage, my salary brings in significantly less than Jamie's, so it's his bonus I'm using— money that we should save, seeing as we are almost always living paycheck to paycheck.

If roles were reversed, and Jamie did such a thing, I'd balk. But he doesn't. He asks, calmly, how I'm going to pay for the trip, and I say that I'm going to ask for donations in lieu of Christmas gifts, though I know full well that no one is going to give me the three grand that the trip will cost when I factor in the flight, hotel, and retreat tuition.

Beyond this one question, Jamie stays silent. Maybe he thinks that if he says anything, I'll snap. And maybe he's right, but, mentally, I justify the trip: I don't have expensive vices or hobbies. In fact, thanks to my money-conscious upbringing and broke grad-school days, I'm more frugal than most. Usually Jamie has to talk me into buying new bras when my ancient Victoria's Secrets disintegrate in the dryer.

And, frankly, haven't I already paid for this trip—not in money, but in myself? Subconsciously, my mind compiles a list that I will lay out for Jamie if he complains about expenses. I realize that because this tally sheet is so readily available in my mind, I must be holding on to some long stuffed-away hurt—hurt that wasn't exposed until my emergency surgery.

"Do you know how much I have sacrificed?" I will ask. Then I will list my sufferings—everything from leaving my life in Chicago, to living in a lonely town, to the endless early-morning IVF appointments, to my emergency surgery, to my scar. Though some of these were my own choices and none were Jamie's fault, they still feel like a penance I've done.

"Surely," I will say, *"I have paid my way."*

Chapter

15

I spend the next three months of winter dodging the one question everyone keeps asking: *When are you going to try IVF again?* Jamie is the only person who doesn't ask me this. Most nights, he sits quietly in his recliner, searching my face to see what's going on in my brain. He knows that I am on the verge of something drastic, that if I don't do something positive *for* myself, I will do something negative *to* myself. He sees my constant preoccupation, how my fear of dying encroaches every day at dusk. He knows that the tradeoff for my typical energetic existence is that my highs are high and my lows are low. But for the first time, I'm unable to reverse the trajectory of my plummeting mood through exercise or journaling, and we're in uncharted territory. He hugs me and holds me. He calls me "sweet girl"—my most favorite nickname. But he and I both know that no amount of his love can fix the quaking in my brain. Only I can repair myself. I just don't know how.

The embryo storage bills continue to come, and we pay them, but I don't want to think about those nine little beings or the Vitello bib in my drawer. I can't even look at the red sharps container from my October injections. Just thinking about needles and ultrasound wands makes me shudder.

The only thing I allow myself to think about is Guatemala.

And then, before I know it, I am sitting in a cab, being sped through the dilapidated streets of Guatemala City.

Sandy and Kate—the two writing-retreat participants I met at the airport—bounce around the cab with me, just hoping to make it to our hotel in one piece.

The driver swerves and races around pickup trucks that puff black exhaust. In the passenger seat, Sandy speaks to him in broken Spanish. She is a middle-aged businesswoman who writes entertaining stories about surviving junior high. Kate and I sit in back, sandwiched by luggage. Unlike straitlaced Sandy, Kate is twenty-two and the essence of quirky. With dyed-blonde hair and eyes that look like a cat's, she's skinny and wiry and shaky with energy. She talks in a honey-sweet voice, and for some reason I can't explain, she's incredibly endearing.

There's a dirty blanket on the seat that Kate fingers instinctively. God only knows where the blanket has been, but Kate looks like she'll nuzzle into it at any second.

After being jolted and jostled around for an hour, we finally arrive in Antigua.

Antigua looks exactly like its name, like something preserved. It's as if the three volcanoes that surround the town are protecting it from modern influence. Stucco colonial buildings painted blue and yellow line cobblestone streets. Even the ruins of the old buildings look like an artist-produced backdrop. Flowers vine around every wall of our hotel, and birds flit through the open-air courtyard to perch on the bubbling fountain.

Here, it's Semana Santa, and the residents parade through the narrow streets carrying crosses and religious relics while they sing and chant. In addition to the holy atmosphere that seeps into my skin via osmosis, we eat dinner in a former convent, and the place is lit entirely by candles that flicker from hidden nooks. Because I spent kindergarten through senior year at Catholic schools, I tend to question the scripture that the nuns forced upon us, but here, I open myself to the sacred aura of it all.

When we sit around with the other women during dinner in the convent, Kate calls me "Pop-Tart" and "cupcake" and nestles into my shoulder like a sibling. She is tender and sarcastic all at once. Our instantaneous friendship feels both easy and fulfilling. I think it's because she embodies all that I have been missing for the last three and a half years—a mother, a sister, a friend.

It feels like no coincidence that only women applied for this retreat. The twelve of us range in age from twenty-two to sixty, from hippie to high maintenance, and yet, it works. In each of these women, I find a Chicago counterpart. Becky is like my always-laughing Grandma Kenney. Molly has Courtney's free spirit. Michelle listens the way Marie does. Sandy has Katy's determination. Christine is shy yet smart, like Jenny. Carol has the same wise gaze as Mom. And Kate is a quirky, extroverted version of Dana. I knew I was coming here for the sun and for the inspiration, but I had no idea that I'd find friendship too.

In high school, I'd wandered from group to group, never feeling fully myself among any clique, but when I went to college, I found that group of funny girls who laughed about the same things I did. Jamie always jokes about secret handshakes and naked pillow fights when I mention my sorority. But living in the sorority was actually this—my friends and I hanging out in sweats on Sundays, talking and laughing, eating dinner together and studying for exams, getting annoyed and bickering yet accepting each other all the same.

If I had the gift of time reversal, there are two time periods I'd go back to—the year I fell in love with Jamie, and the year I lived in that sorority with my friends. But because I can't go back, I'll take this altered version of a sorority dinner—sitting around a long wooden table in the converted convent while the candles flicker and women from all over the country share their stories. "Cheers, cupcake," Kate says, and I clink my glass with hers. Someone tells a joke, and the table erupts. We wipe our eyes and agree that women's laughter might be the loveliest sound in all the world.

The next day, our two instructors—my friends Jenn and Adam from Boston—lead us on a three-hour bus trip to Panajachel, where we board a water shuttle to take us to the retreat.

We ride the rocky boat into the fog, the volcanoes and shoreline only half-visible through the mist, and we're so low in the lake and so blindfolded by cloudy air that I feel like I am heading to the end of the earth. Soon, the water will drop off, and we will float into some kind of kingdom that awaits us.

The fog evaporates and what lies ahead does, actually, resemble a heavenly empire—a dock, twinkle lights, a large house with walls of windows, a terraced lawn of gardens, a veranda with wooden patio furniture, and two lake-view guesthouses. Our retreat leader, Joyce, stands on the dock, bedazzled in blue, and welcomes us.

I am sure there are more luxurious places on this earth, but I don't want them. I'll take this. I'll take this any day.

At night, we eat chicken and asparagus on the patio as the water laps and the moon climbs up the volcano. Then Joyce gives us gifts—thick, soft shawls of different colors. Mine is blue, my favorite hue. I wrap it around my shoulders and my eyes tear. I feel full. I feel fed. I feel warmed. I feel loved. Mom and Dana and my friends are woven into the threads of the shawl and they are hugging me tight. They are squeezing me.

They are forgiving me for neglecting them when I moved. They are saying, "You deserve this self-repair. You deserve to be in the healing company of women."

Kate, who's cloaked in a green shawl, sees me dabbing at my eyes.

"I'm just really, really happy," I tell her.

"I know. It's so nice, isn't it?" she says. I don't know if she's talking about the shawl, or the place, or both.

Later, when we take the boat to our new hotel, the moon is so huge and reflective that it feels like it is dipping down into the lake and kissing me with its light.

The town we're staying in—San Marcos—is new-age naturalist meets Mayan medicine man. Dirt paths weave through junglelike landscapes and emerge at outdoor yoga centers and massage huts and meditation spots. The place is full of toking ex-pats and locals in traditional garb. Outnumbering the people, stray dogs wander around the bodegas and churches until someone shoos them away. Roosters and birds sing constantly, and creatures scurry in the dirt. The air smells of burning campfires.

San Marcos is shaped like a guitar pick, with two sides bordered by the waters of Lake Atitlan. In the morning, I walk to Joyce's house. Beyond her iron gate and gardens, her dock juts out over the water. Joyce invited us all to join her for a ritual morning swim, but Becky and I are the only ones who woke up early enough.

I'm nervous. Not because I'm diving into a large, deep lake, but because I am wearing a two-piece for the first time since my surgery. There's no denying my scar. Its dark line runs from my belly button to my bikini bottoms. It appears darker in some spots than others and forces my ab muscles to bulge more on the left.

Wrapped in my towel, I follow the women onto the dock.

As we stand there, about to jump in, I squirm internally, not wanting to disrobe. *I look like a freak,* I think. *My stomach resembles an awful stitching project.* Becky and Joyce discuss the best way to get in, and there's no other option than to disrobe and dive. So, I unravel my towel and place it on the dock. Becky feigns polite ignorance, but Joyce asks about my scar right away. After we dive into the cool water, we paddle, and I tell them my story.

"We have nine frozen embryos in storage," I say as I breaststroke in circles. "They told me I could try again six weeks after the surgery, but I just wasn't ready. I mean, my body recovered, but mentally, I'm just not . . . I wasn't there." I find myself struggling with the verb tense, like I'm in the middle of getting there, but I haven't yet arrived.

The women nod, not needing an explanation.

"You should write about those babies," Joyce says.

And this is another first: the first time anyone has ever referred to our embryos as babies.

Every morning after our swim, Joyce, Becky, and I rinse off under the outdoor shower on Joyce's balcony, then we head downstairs for breakfast. Each day, the cook prepares a buffet of garlicky eggs, tortillas, black beans, cheese, yogurt, fresh mango, banana, strong coffee, and cream. The other women usually arrive just as the food is served and we sit around the small patio tables, chirping along with the birds. The sun dries my dripping hair as I laugh and refill my plate.

Once our bellies are full, we head to a thatched-roof section of lawn where we workshop stories. I've brought parts of my novel to be discussed, and during our breaks, I write ferociously, as if there are volumes of words inside of me just waiting to break out. At lunch, we head to town for avocados or go for a swim. I find myself proud to wear my bikini now and openly tell the other women about my scar. Then we spend the afternoon back under the thatched roof for more writing discussions until it's time for dinner and wine. As the sun sets, we play games and laugh and eat and drink, then head upstairs to the large sitting room, where we snuggle up on a long red couch and read our work aloud.

At around nine, we ride the boat back to our hotel under the light of the looming moon. Then, once docked, we find our way to our rooms by flashlight. Kate and Molly climb up to my rooftop balcony with me and we stay up chatting for hours.

I fall asleep each night so full of contentment that my heart might burst. My muscles ache from all the walking, my cheeks from all the laughing. I've written more stories in three days than I have in six months. I've never felt so happily exhausted.

Midweek, we get a free afternoon, and a few of us decide to hike up to a mountain peak called La Nariz.

No problem, I think, *I'll get some good exercise and a great view.* But our two local teenage guides scurry up the hillside before I can even get my footing. Kate and Molly follow closely behind. I can't keep up with them, and I reason it's because they're five years younger than I am. But then Michelle, who's my age, joins their group and keeps pace, while I fall to the back of the pack with Sandy on my right and Becky on my left. Though they are great company, they're twenty years my senior, so my stamina should be slightly better than theirs. *Why can't I keep up with the younger girls?* I wonder. *The Chicago marathon wasn't even this hard.* But, still, my quads ache and my lungs burn. I have to take breaks—panting, bent-over breaks. I don't like taking breaks. I am not a break taker. But my lungs and my legs tell me that I must. And so it goes—I climb, I stop. I climb, I stop. I climb, I stop. In order to resist giving up, I keep my eye on the peak. Every step closer fuels me to keep going.

We hike through a forest, then a hillside farm, then an almost-vertical incline, and, finally, we clamber onto a wooden lookout where we take in the view—the glorious sky and volcanoes and lake. It is the tropical version of Maine: water surrounded by green peaks. And I'm on top of it all. I pause to inhale the moment. It fills me until I expand into the air molecules around me. I feel large enough to leap from one volcano to the next. I could slide down their sides and into the glimmering pool below.

Molly, Kate, Michelle, and I stretch into yoga postures on the wooden platform, and I get the sensation that I am doing cobra pose on the clouds. I'm proud of myself for completing the hike, even though the journey wasn't pretty. My body folds into child's pose, surrendering.

After an hour on the wooden platform, a van is supposed to pick us up, but it doesn't come. From the guides' rapid Spanish, I don't understand if the van isn't working or their cell phones aren't, but we start descending on foot. We walk and we walk. My frustration grows. We've been hiking and walking for hours, and we should already be back at our hotel, where I had planned to treat myself to some sunbathing and writing—a rare gift, because if I were back in Massachusetts, at the university, I'd be teaching my fourth class of the day.

Now I feel the way I felt when I woke up in the hospital in October—frustrated that life has interrupted my plans and that there is nothing I can do about it. But the guides don't seem at all worried or apologetic. They just keep walking past farms and hut-houses, past a skinny guy and his skinny horse both carrying such heavy stacks of wood on their backs that it's a surprise they're not collapsing. I feel like a jerk, but I'm still sour as we stop on side of the road.

We wait and wait and wait.

Michelle, a California girl who moved here for her Gua-

temalan husband, says that this is normal. This is Guatemalan
time. Things happen when they happen.

I don't like Guatemalan time. But what choice do I have?

Then, a rickety pickup squeals to a stop at our feet, and
our guides encourage us to join the locals who stand in the bed
of the truck. This will be our ride back. Michelle hops on like
it's nothing. Here, she explains, pickup trucks are like cabs—
you can pay the driver to take you where you need to go. So,
we all pile in. The bed of the truck is so heavy it almost scrapes
the tires, and we grip a waist-high bar for support. The truck
speeds down the winding hillside. Even though I'm partly terrified of falling to my death, I love feeling the wind in my hair,
and it seems that the other women do, too. We laugh like
we're on a roller coaster.

The truck deposits us in another town where we hail tuk-
tuks, little golf-cart vehicles, that zoom us back to our hotel.

"Well," I say as we pay the driver, "that wasn't exactly how
I was expecting to get back."

Those words stick with me as I sit on my hotel balcony
mulling things over—this day, this year. I lift up my shirt, feeling the wrinkled skin of my scar, warmed now by the healing
sun. I look up at the sky and think, *OK, up there, whoever you
are—supreme ruler, master of the universe, higher power—I get it. I
get the symbolism, I get the message. Maybe, this isn't how I expected
IVF to go, but I have to keep pressing forward, and eventually, I'll get
there.*

Some way, somehow, I will have a baby.

On the last day of the retreat, the instructors give us a
parting gift—a journal with a woven cover that says Guatemala. We cuddle up on the long red couch and watch a slide
show of pictures from the week, then we reminisce and hug
each other goodbye. It feels like a graduation. I am almost
afraid to go back to the real world because my time here has

been so sacred. But the good news is that Kate lives in Massachusetts, as do Jenn and Adam, and I plan to see them often.

At the airport, I feel lost wandering around by myself. Kate arrived here earlier because her flight leaves before mine, and our gates are at opposite ends of the airport. When I go through security, I see her green shawl in the left-behind pile at the screening checkpoint. Using my broken Spanish, I communicate to the guard that the shawl is my friend's, and I search the monitors until I find her gate. Kate is pretzeled in a seat and going through her carry-on bag. When I sit down next to her and present her with the shawl, she squeals and lights up.

"Thanks, Pop-Tart," she says as she hugs me.

The flight attendant announces the boarding call, and Kate wraps her shawl around her shoulders, then grabs her bag.

"You and me," she says, "writing date next week. Promise?"

"Sounds good," I say, excited about Saturday afternoons of writing and coffee drinking that will no longer be solitary.

After watching her blonde hair and green shawl disappear through the doors, I turn, smiling, to walk to my gate.

In a private seat in the corner, I spread my blue shawl over my now-tan legs. For the next hour, I fill page after page of my new Guatemala journal with memories from the trip. My hope is that capturing them will continue the self-healing that I started in this magical place.

When Jamie picks me up at the airport, he squeezes me as if we've been apart for years. We are so happy to see each other, we can't stop kissing and intertwining our fingers the whole ride home. "When you were away," he says, "it felt like we were divorced or something. It was so lonely." And I realize that this is what IVF can do to people. Rather than needing a week away, some people might get so overwhelmed that they need a complete separation.

At a red light, I tap Jamie's arm so that he'll look me in the eye. "Thank you," I tell him. "Thank you for knowing how much I needed this."

"You're welcome," he says.

Over the next few weeks, Jamie writes me cards almost daily, reaches for me every chance he gets. In turn, I write him lovey emails, hug him for no reason. He looks at me with his crooked smile, like I am the most perfect woman on the planet.

The forsythia in our neighborhood blooms, announcing spring, and I find myself grinning for no reason during drives and jogs. I meet up with Kate for writing dates, with Jenn for coffee. Even the Facebook communication with the women I met on the retreat brings me daily joy.

Back in October, I couldn't have imagined ever being ready to try IVF again, but Guatemala and spring and friendship and Jamie's extra love have all nourished me back to health.

One April evening, I open my drawer and fish through my camisoles until my fingers grasp the strings of our Vitello bib. I bring it to my chest for a hug.

When Jamie and I spoon in bed that night, I whisper to him, "Let's talk to the doctor."

He kisses the back of my neck and pulls me closer.

"You're ready?" he asks gently.

"I'm ready," I say.

Chapter

1 6

Per Joyce's suggestion, I start thinking about our nine frozen embryos as our children.

I name them, envision their personalities.

Geo is a future astrologist, Raya perks up in the afternoon, Caleb hates mashed peas, Jinny sucks her pinkies, Ariana is nearsighted, Ty prefers to be alone, Percy plays with his belly button, Will has a slight lisp, and Lucy wears glittery shoes.

I imagine that they look like miniature toddlers swimming inside ice cubes. In fact, nowadays, I only fill nine squares of our ice tray. Every night before dinner, I plunk four cubes into Jamie's glass, five into mine. I like to think that our whole brood is with us at the table, comparing stories from the day.

Of course, I'd never confess this ice cube–children idea to anyone. I hope that this is what other IVF women do, too— imagine, fantasize, develop eyebrow-raising rituals.

It's late afternoon and Jamie and I sit on the plaid couch in our sunroom as dusk sneaks in through our bamboo blinds. Jamie lies across the sofa, his legs draped over the armrest, his head in my lap, and I massage his scalp down to the collar of his unbuttoned work shirt.

Tomorrow we have an appointment with our reproductive specialist to discuss the process of transferring one of the embryos into my uterus. Jamie says how lucky we are to have nine chances at getting pregnant. I hold on to this number, wear it on my finger like a diamond. *Nine,* oh how it sparkles.

Jamie takes a sip of his iced tea, then rests it on his stomach. The ice cubes are melting, turning the brown liquid into a soft amber, but I'm reassured that our actual babies are in a temperature-controlled home, protected from liquefying, from evaporating. I envision them in an aquarium-like tank, floating around, safe in their respective ice blocks. Raya zooms around in her dice of ice, while Geo drifts lazily.

Jamie closes his eyes when I scratch his scalp. We talk about the embryo transfer, and I list worries that begin with "what if" and end in "miscarriage," in "birth defect." Jamie opens his eyes, pulls my face down toward his. He kisses me perpendicularly and his stubble rubs my nose.

"We have nine tries," he says. "One of them has to take."

When the room turns gray, it's time to prepare dinner.

Tessa prefers frozen broccoli over kibble, so I pour some icy florets into her dish. We're out of fresh greens, and I consider using some of the broccoli to accompany the cod we're eating. But I hate how even after cooking frozen veggies, there's still the metallic remains of freezer burn, the aftertaste of the other items—like Hot Pockets and breakfast sausages— that pressed against it in the freezer.

I wonder—*Will our sons and daughters be different because they were frozen? Will they have brains that are mushy from thawing? Will they behave less vibrantly than a naturally conceived child? Will they smell faintly of ground turkey?*

The next day, we arrive at the headquarters grinning but

clasping each other's hands tightly. A pregnant nurse escorts us to the doctor's office, her belly protruding so much that she can't button the bottom of her white coat. I must resist the urge to prod, the way I did with our specialist, and find out if it's an IVF baby.

Jamie asks the nurse where our babies are being stored, but "stored" seems like the wrong word, as if they're stacked in cardboard boxes, getting dusty at a warehouse. I hadn't thought about the fact that our little gang is in this very building. I want to visit them the way one might stop by a hospital nursery, peering at them through the glass—chubby legs in blue and pink socks, gummy mouths cooing and drooling.

The nurse rubs her belly, then points down a hallway with paintings of flowers that resemble vaginas. "The cryo lab is down there."

"Are the embryos kept in ice cube trays?" I half-joke.

She laughs and says no; they're actually in thin tubes. "Like coffee stirrers," she says.

"How big are they?" I ask.

"Smaller than a pin head."

Jamie's eyes widen as mine squint with disappointment. He whispers, "That's unbelievable."

Our doctor welcomes us into her office. I haven't seen her since she came to my hospital room and announced that the extraction needles might have been too sharp. She looks even skinnier, her cheekbones even more severe. Though she is not the doctor who performed that actual egg retrieval, I still feel uneasy around her and worry that she wasn't conservative enough with my injection doses, which may have led to an excess of eggs in my ovaries. Jamie and I talked at length about switching clinics. But, ultimately, we agreed that it was in our best interest to stay. If we go to another clinic, we have to start all over again and repeat tests we've already taken. But the major deterrent against switching is that, if we go to another clinic, we risk something happening to our embryos when they're being transported. If our embryos didn't survive the journey to their new office, I'd have to do the injections and the egg retrieval all over again. And I am not willing to risk the same procedure that nearly killed me.

But if we stay at this clinic, where our embryos are, I can progress to the next step—the transfer—without any fuss. The procedure is so quick that I'm not even sedated for it. Plus, I've already requested that the doctor who did my egg retrieval not be allowed anywhere near me.

As usual, our specialist is drinking Diet Coke through a bendy straw.

After she explains how we'll prep my body, she asks how many embryos we want to transfer. Back in the fall, we were going to transfer two, but now that I've been through hospital hell, I want to be more careful with my body.

"One," I say. "We'll save the rest so we can have more children later. I don't want to transfer them all at once. I have no desire to be the next Octomom."

"You can't exactly assume that you'll have extra embryos," the doctor says.

"Why is that?" Jamie asks. He shifts in his chair, reaches over, places his hand in mine.

The doctor takes another sip of her Diet Coke and says, "Well, they have to survive the thaw."

Jamie's voice is steady, but his cheeks flush. "What is the survival rate?"

"Fifty-fifty," she says, not looking at us.

I grip Jamie's hand.

Caleb and Jinny and Ariana and Ty and Lucy melt in my mind.

"So, hypothetically speaking," Jamie says, "we have four

potential babies."

"Not necessarily." She explains how the next hurdle is that they have to attach to the uterine wall.

"Only about 30 percent of thawed embryos take to the womb," she says.

Will and Percy and Raya dissolve into puddles. Only Geo is left.

"But if you transfer two," the doctor says, "you raise your chances." She throws her now-empty can into the garbage. "Then again, you could always end up with twins."

Raya resolidifies.

"Well, that's not the end of the world," Jamie says, turning toward me. "We could get our family out of the way in one swoop."

"Yes," the doctor says, "but you also have to consider that they most likely won't reach full gestation. All twins, IVF or not, are typically born early."

The room is quiet, and I bite my nails.

"So, you have a decision to make," the doctor says. "If more than one embryo survives the thaw, do you want to transfer one or two?"

That night when I pull out the ice cube tray to fill our glasses, I can no longer envision the squares as our children or even as embryos. They are crystallized water. They are not swimming around. They do not have names. They do not have personalities. We don't know if any will endure the great defrost, and if they do, we can't control if any will be strong enough to hold on once inside.

I turn the tray over, twist it a bit, and let the frosty contents fall into the sink. Lines shoot up the center of the cubes, crevasses forming.

Just as I'm about to leave the cubes to drip and drain, I peer down and examine them closely. Some are chipped at the edges, but most of them are still intact, still solid. They are not as fragile as I thought.

I pick the two without cracks and gently slip them into my glass.

My brain wants to protect my heart by saying *if*: *If* the embryos survive. *If* I get pregnant. But now, just a few weeks before our frozen embryo transfer, I'm vibrating with positive energy. I'm trying to use the word *if* less. Last time we didn't tell our friends and family about IVF, for fear of jinxing the whole thing. But that obviously didn't prevent horrible things from happening. So, when we do the embryo transfer, I'm going to announce the good news to everyone.

My gut says that we *are* going to be successful. Out of our nine frozen babies, and the two that we will transfer—Geo and Raya—I think, for some reason, that Geo is going to survive. He will be the same blonde-haired, blue-eyed boy I've been envisioning ever since I first fell in love with Jamie six years ago and saw the framed photo of him as a baby. *Geo,* I say to myself, *short for George the fifth.* G.E.O. Our Earth. Our World.

I've been reading IVF discussion forums and blog posts, and I'm relieved to know that I am not alone in the fantasizing and naming of unborn children. It seems that, for those of us who want children badly or have suffered through IVF, visualization is the thing that keeps us going. It is our form of a positive affirmation. Our belief is that the more we think about our babies, the more likely the universe will bring them to us.

In the morning, when I make lunches for Jamie, I doodle sketches and stick them on his packets of oatmeal, his baggies of almonds. I draw Jamie pushing Geo's stroller, Jamie giving Geo and Tessa a bath, Jamie carrying Geo in a BabyBjörn and teaching him how to make his famous home fries for breakfast. When I go to yoga on a warm night at the end of April, positivity radiates from my pores. I don't care that I won't be able to do my heated classes after the end of this month, because all that matters is we are going to have a successful transfer.

Tonight, after class, I wait for all the sweaty yogis to leave the humid studio, and I approach the front desk to tell Linda that I have to cancel my monthly membership.

She looks through my file, says that I can't terminate it until after June without being penalized.

"It's for medical reasons," I explain, taking my hair out of its bun. "We're doing our embryo transfer in a few weeks, and I can't do hot yoga once I'm pregnant." I'm pleased with myself for not saying, "*If* we're fortunate enough to become pregnant . . ."

I'm excited to continue the conversation Linda and I started six months ago, when she hinted that she had used fertility treatments. Instead of giving me an encouraging smile, she averts her gaze, then creases the corner of my membership contract. I stare at her bandanna, wondering why she won't look me in the eye.

"Have you ever done a transfer?" she asks, still not looking up.

I shake my head no. She nods and closes the file folder.

"You must have done one, right," I ask, "seeing as you have a daughter?"

"Oh, I did a lot of transfers, and I got pregnant from them," she says, "but I always miscarried. After all that IVF shit," she adds, breaking her yogic calmness, "I ended up taking Clomid and got pregnant just like that." She snaps her fingers.

My sweat, now cool, goose-bumps my skin.

She asks me to keep talking to her while she goes back in the studio, and as she douses the hard wood with vinegar, I stand in the doorway. She pushes around the mop and tells me how her ex's sperm swam backward, how they had years of infertility, and how they divorced just a few years after her daughter was born.

"Five years of infertility," she says. "And we never talked about it. All that shit can really build up."

When I leave the studio, the warm spring night has cooled off, and it shivers my skin. The *ifs* are back. *What if this transfer doesn't work? What if I bleed internally again?*

I sit in my car thinking about it all. *How do two people go through all of those losses, only to get divorced?* I wonder. *Were the cracks in their marriage there even before, or did IVF cause them? And what about Jamie and me? Surely this has put stress on our relationship. But it would never split us apart. Right?*

I make a choice to boycott all the IVF books, websites, discussion forums, and blogs I've been perusing. Now that I'm weighed down with Linda's story and those I've read on the blogs, I don't want to hear the war stories anymore.

Sure, it's comforting to know that these women also struggled through hormone boot camp, that they stabbed and injected their own flesh nightly, waited for test results, reenlisted time and again. But, finally, they received and proudly displayed their badges in the form of wrinkled newborns.

These women eventually bore children, *after* three failed IVF cycles, *after* eight miscarriages.

I don't know anymore if I'm cut out for this, if I'm capable of witnessing the casualties without going crazy.

A couple days later, while at Panera doing work, I open an email from Jamie's cousin, Amy. She's a birth coach who knows about our fertility struggles.

Her email starts off this way: *You will get pregnant. Of this much I am sure.*

No one has said this to us. Not the doctors, not our friends. Jamie and I haven't even said this to ourselves, at least not with this much certainty. She writes that I should try envisioning the baby growing in my womb.

This helps me realize something: I've sketched Geo. I've sketched Tess and Geo. I've sketched Jamie and Tess and Geo, but I've never drawn myself with a belly bump, or with Geo in my arms.

So I take out my journal and start drawing. Even though my self-portrait is a poorly sketched stick figure with long hair, and my baby bump looks more like an ulcer, it seems just a tad more possible that this *will* be me in the future. In the very near future.

Chapter

17

Estrogen is a bitch.

It makes me hormonal, and I cry in the shower for no reason. But what really concerns me is that I've had the same throbbing headache on the back left side of my skull for four days straight and the vision in my left eye is getting blurrier by the day. Jamie and I are due to have our embryo transfer in just two weeks. I could be pregnant in fourteen short days. I want to suck it up and suffer through the hormone hell so that we can complete the cycle.

If I complain to the clinic too much, our cycle might be canceled. We'd have to start this process all over again. I'm so sick of having my life paused and rewound by IVF. I'm sick of the waiting and the not knowing. It's hard to even remember what life was like when babies and estrogen levels weren't a constant preoccupation.

But the headaches and the blurriness persist, and because the IVF books have mentioned patients getting blood clots from the estrogen, I fear for my health. *How far am I willing to go?* I ask myself one night as my head throbs. *How much of myself am I willing to sacrifice for the possibility of getting pregnant?*

The next morning, I call the nurses, and they switch me from estrogen pills to a patch. Still, with each passing day, my symptoms persist. So, I call them and visit my primary care doctor.

They give me the following responses:

Fertility Nurse #1: It's just a side effect of the hormones. Sometimes women get really bad migraines after an influx of estrogen.

PCP: Hmmm, it could be a sinus infection.

Fertility Nurse #2: Women rarely complain about side effects with the estrogen patch. Your symptoms might not be related at all. Maybe it's your glasses or your contacts. I'd visit your eye doctor.

PCP: You know, based on your symptoms, there's always the possibility of shingles.

Fertility Nurse #3: Have you been drinking enough water? Maybe you're just dehydrated.

PCP: We also have to consider Lyme disease. Or Bell's palsy. This might be the early stages of Bell's palsy.

Then, after class one afternoon, as my last student leaves, I check my voicemail. Fertility Nurse #4 says, "Take the estrogen patch off immediately. We're concerned that you could have a blood clot. This could be potentially life-threatening. We need to stop the cycle."

I stand in my empty classroom listening to the last message over and over again. Students spill out of other classrooms, heading home, and I wait for the hallway to clear. On autopilot, my arms gather my books and student essays. My legs walk to the faculty bathroom. My hands close the stall door. My fingers peel off the patch and drop it into the garbage. My brain lists the pros and cons of my next steps:

Do another cycle; risk a blood clot.

Switch clinics; risk the embryos dying during transportation.

Try conceiving naturally; risk never getting pregnant.

A sentence scribbles across my brain, unable to be erased: We. Have. No. Options.

Once I'm off the estrogen patch, my headaches subside and my vision normalizes. Was there a blood clot? We'll never know. The whole incident is just as mysterious as everything else that has happened. But I'm not the only one whom medicine isn't helping. Grandma Kenney, ridden with ALS, is deteriorating quickly. Two weeks after our canceled cycle, when Jamie and I are in Chicago for a friend's wedding, we drive out to the suburbs to visit her.

Grandma's little house looks the same, with a blooming garden by her back door and birdhouses hanging around the patio. So I imagine that she'll look the same as well—running to the door wearing her usual capris and nylons. Her hair will be dyed a sandy blonde and her eyebrows will be precisely drawn. She'll greet us with tea and her award-winning Irish bread.

But when we knock at the slider, she staggers to the door. Her mouth hangs open; drool collects in the corners. A lead weight, her left arm seems dead. She has lost thirty pounds, and her skin sags off of her bones. She is mute minus a moan. When we hug, her right arm—her good arm—grips me so tightly it's like she's begging to be rescued.

As usual, every inch of her house is adorned with pictures, fake flowers, lace curtains, antiques. But now, her cloth bouquets are crowded by breathing machines and cans of feeding-tube formula. There are vials upon vials of medicine—the only things keeping her alive.

It isn't ALS that kills people—it's the pneumonia that sets in, or the malnourishment, or, simply, the inability to breathe.

Grandma Kenney shuffles over to her armchair and takes out her whiteboard. Putting a paper towel up to her mouth, she lets her drool dampen it and uses that to wipe off the marker. "How my hony?" she writes. I don't know if she's always had trouble spelling or if this is something recent.

"Who, me?" I ask, but she points at Jamie. Ever since she met him, Grandma has designated Jamie her honey.

She writes things on her whiteboard slowly, forgetting words and letters, but we do our best to comprehend. I tell her story after story so she doesn't feel bad about being unable to talk. She moans, nods her head.

Grandma has a quarter lung capacity left, and still, Grandpa enters the room with a cigarette dangling from his mouth. He heads outside and props a ladder against the house. On her whiteboard, Grandma urges Jamie to help him.

My aunt and I try to fill the room with more talk, but, instead, I'm staring at this unrecognizable version of my grandmother. Her hair is platinum blonde. She definitely left the Nice 'n Easy in for too long. I think about how hard it must have been to wash it out with only one working hand. She has whiskers on her upper lip I've never seen before and her legs are bare. I'm guessing nylons are too tiresome to put on. Like tattoos covering her ankles, her varicose veins are deep green and thick.

I have the urge to wash her hair, dye it the right shade, pluck her whiskers, and help her into her nylons, even if that means seeing her naked body and the feeding tube protruding from her abdomen. Instead, I sit on the arm of her chair and caress her right bicep. She's so thin that there's no muscle tone, and it feels like I'm rubbing a deflated balloon.

A cup of tea sits cold on the side table. She never once sips from it, and I wonder if she just makes it out of habit.

Jamie returns, having cleaned out the gutters—a project Grandpa's been working on for three days.

When Grandma blinks heavily, it's time to leave.

She walks to the kitchen and shows us a lovely brown loaf of Irish bread she baked for us. I almost break down right then. I don't know how she made it, working with just one hand. I don't even know how she lifted it out of the oven.

What makes me sadder, though, is the realization that she can't eat it—this food she loves so much. If she does, she'll choke. Sensing my questions, she writes something on her whiteboard, and I can't make it out, but my aunt translates.

"I taste."

Before we head out, we take pictures that I know I won't be able to look at later. The flash captures a skinny, lopsided woman that is not my grandmother. When we say goodbye, she cries silently in her armchair, mouth agape. I try to comfort her, but she writes on her whiteboard: "Go."

So we leave.

After the wedding, back in Massachusetts, I freeze the hunk of Irish bread that Grandma gave us.

A week later, she dies.

I give the eulogy at her funeral in Illinois, while, in Massachusetts, my sister-in-law celebrates her baby shower. She and Josh are having a little girl, whom they're going to name Lily.

After we fly from Chicago back to Boston, we stop at Jamie's parents' house on our drive home from the airport. We stand around the island and talk for a while, then Judi shows us a card and explains that, at Ciara's baby shower, everyone received a blank note to fill out for one of Lily's future birthdays.

She hands me the card for Lily's eighth birthday so that we can write a message on it. Hives blotch my chest and I try to pick up the pen, but my fingers refuse to grip it. I have to excuse myself to the bathroom. My logical brain knows that we should fill out the card and hand it back to Judi, but none of the pep talks I give myself in the bathroom mirror make me want to go out there and pick up that pen. Our canceled transfer and the loss of Grandma Kenney have left me empty, and I can siphon not a single drop of strength from the dry well in my soul.

When I emerge from the bathroom, I see that Jamie hasn't touched the card either. "We'll fill it out later," I say and slip it in my purse. Judi's eyes search our faces, and upon registering our pain, she opens the refrigerator and looks for something to feed us. I feel bad that she is caught in the middle of being sad for one son and happy for the other, but it still doesn't make my envy go away.

A couple days later, in my own private memorial to Grandma Kenney, I defrost a piece of her loaf. As it warms in the toaster oven, nutmeg and cinnamon fill the air. More than any perfume, these are the smells that conjure her, and I imagine her sitting at our dining room table with me, eating the way she used to—loud and openmouthed, as if she was always mid-laugh.

I think about how Grandma spent the time she was sick—still baking, still tasting food even when she couldn't swallow it. She wanted other people to enjoy eating her Irish bread even though she couldn't. I think about how I'm spending my time—in jealousy, in fear. But what if we try another cycle and it puts my life in danger again? We're stuck. We can't conceive naturally or artificially. What other options do we have?

I take another bite of bread and wonder if our infertility will be incurable, like Grandma's ALS.

"Get another opinion," my mind tells me.

It's the only real option—to find a different doctor—but it requires work.

There are so many hurdles: doing the research, reading the reviews, getting the insurance approval, moving our embryos.

"OK, then do nothing," my mind says. *"How has that been working out for you?"*

We need to do something, anything. If we don't, I will live the rest of my life with the void of a baby who is so vibrant in my mind that I can smell his skin as clearly as I can taste the bread on my tongue.

So I put the last sweet morsels of nutmeg and raisin into my mouth and make a promise to call at least one new doctor today.

Then I sit there, chewing the bread.

Tasting it.

Our new fertility specialist is Dr. Peters. He has a completely different approach than our former doctor. He always airs on the conservative side. He's more thorough, more patient, and because he operates out of the same headquarters as our previous specialist, we don't have to risk transporting our embryos.

Even his office has a completely different vibe. It's bright and welcoming, with pictures of former patients' kids. Our three-inch file rests on his desk, open, and it seems he has combed through every page. He notices something that the other doctor never mentioned. Although Jamie's sperm showed low motility and morphology in a couple of tests, Jamie's counts in October, when he gave the sperm that fertilized our embryos, were much closer to normal. Dr. Peters encourages Jamie to have his sperm tested again because if the results are better, we might not need the doctor's help at all.

We cross our fingers, and Jamie gives another sample.

What if? I think. *What if Jamie's sperm wasn't as compromised as we'd thought?*

The regret-filled road is treacherous to navigate, but I traverse it anyway.

Would we have avoided all of this trauma if we had just tried for longer on our own? Would we have a naturally conceived newborn right now?

For a couple weeks, I'm like the rest of the smiling population, enjoying the summertime, feeling hopeful. Jamie and I eat dinner on our porch, listening to the crickets. We make love spontaneously.

The next time we meet with Dr. Peters in June, we sit at his desk, excited to receive the results of Jamie's analysis.

But he explains that, unfortunately, Jamie's counts are low again.

Were the October results a fluke? Were they a consequence of certain vitamins or diet choices? We'll never know. But all is not lost. The doctor says we have another option: I can do a natural cycle. Instead of taking estrogen to control my hormones, we'll wait for my own ovulation process and transfer two embryos then. Though this means almost daily blood work, it also means no injections, no headaches, no risk of blood clots. For the transfer procedure, the doctors will insert the embryos into a catheter, which passes through my cervix. Then they'll push liquid down the tube to send the embryos into my uterus. After that, I will have to take progesterone to help things along, but only for the two weeks until my pregnancy test.

I wonder why our other doctor never even revealed that there was a natural option, why she didn't reveal a lot of things. Where would we be right now if we had just gotten a second opinion from the get-go?

But the fact that we have options now and that I won't be a slave to hormones gives us new hope. We leave his office smiling and holding hands. I actually feel eager to move forward, knowing that I won't be putting my own health at risk.

Our new perspective even helps us get through the hardest day of all: getting the call that Ciara is in labor with Lily. Jamie and I gather our things to drive to Maine, where they live, and my mind braces itself for jealousy to barge in, but only excitement enters. Without crying, I'm able to pack Ciara's baby shower gift and buy a dozen bagels for everyone at the hospital.

During the three-hour drive up north, Jamie and I discuss how I, too, might have been giving birth right now *if* my egg-retrieval recovery hadn't gone completely awry. But we also talk about our upcoming natural cycle. It's better for my body and the embryos to follow my own hormone flux rather than that of synthetic injections. It seems fail-proof.

When we arrive in Maine, Lily has just been born and we wait in the hospital's lobby excited. Every time the maternity ward door opens, we look up, expectantly, for Jamie's brother. When he finally emerges, Jamie and I hug each other and head in.

Lily's tiny arms and legs flail on the changing table, and my voice catches in my throat. My cheeks are moist before I even have the chance to reach for a tissue. They are partially tears of longing but mostly tears of possibility.

This is what we can have very soon, I think.

And then I reach out my hands to hold her.

Chapter

18

The luxury of a natural cycle comes with a price. Between the drive to the hospital, the waiting, the blood work, the ultrasounds, and the extra time added to my work commute, the whole process takes two hours out of each day. I am late to class almost every single morning. Any day now, the director is going to walk into my classroom, see all my students waiting there with no teacher in sight, and she's going to fire me.

Also, because I want this cycle to be different, I try every homeopathic method of preparing my uterus lining for babies: eat more flaxseed, drink 100 percent pomegranate juice, go for morning walks to increase blood flow, sustain from alcohol. I am determined to develop a super-womb.

The one time Jamie has to drop off a sperm sample, he complains so fervently about how it's going to interrupt his day that I offer—passive-aggressively—to bring it to the hospital for him.

I want him to say, "*No, I'll do it. It's the least I can do.*" But he doesn't.

I shove the plastic cup into a brown paper bag with such force that Jamie raises his eyebrows.

"What's wrong?" he asks.

"Nothing," I say and slam the door shut as I get into my car and head to the hospital. The sun is barely awake, and I stew the whole drive, thinking, *The one time. The one fucking time you have to do something IVF related, and you complain. This is my life every single day. So, don't you even. Don't you even try to act like it's some major inconvenience. Because you have no fucking idea.*

But I convince myself that stress isn't conducive to a welcoming environment for our embryos. Plus, if I grumble about IVF to Jamie, he'll feel bad about the reason why we have to do IVF. His low sperm motility is an uncontrollable issue, but it still makes him self-conscious. And if I had the guts to just be honest and say that it's really important to me that he drop off the sample himself, I know he would.

The thing is, I could be completely centered, but the moment that anger blinds me, I forget every coping strategy my yoga instructors have ever taught me. I become Mom. But instead of stomping to the bathroom for a smoke like she used to, I ignite an imaginary fight. I inhale all the things that Jamie would say to me, and I exhale all the sharp, cutting lines I would have delivered if I hadn't been so speechless with anger back at our house when he handed me the sample.

By the time my car pulls into the hospital parking lot, I stub it all out. I don't talk with Jamie or anyone else about how the weight of this baby journey is all on my shoulders. I don't ask a single soul for support.

We go in for the long-awaited transfer on a sunny July Saturday nine and a half months after my botched egg retrieval and internal bleeding. But I'm not thinking about the child I could have conceived back then. I'm thinking about the child I'll be conceiving today and delivering nine months from now.

We expect the transfer to be some momentous occasion, but in a matter of thirty minutes, we sign the paperwork and the doctors begin passing a catheter through my cervix to make a gateway for the embryos. The nurses have given me a Valium to relax my uterus muscles, yet the tube does not feel like it's merely "passing through" my cervix. It feels like the time I pierced my own ear by shoving a post through my cartilage.

But the beautiful, unexpected part of the process is that we get to see our embryos under a microscope just before they're injected. Jamie and I decided on two embryos because Dr. Peters said that this would most likely result in a single pregnancy. They look like two flowers with their eight-cell circles, and the nurse gives us a picture of them to put on our refrigerator.

Then, the doctor inserts the embryos into the tube and shoots them into my uterus.

He removes the tube, and we're done.

It seems impossible that the process is that simple.

I lie on the table to let the embryos settle into place while Jamie and I hold up our flower photo and smile. Then we talk to my stomach, addressing our babies.

Jamie leans down to my belly button and says, "Hello in there. This is your dad. Isn't Mom's uterus so nice and cozy? Do us a favor and make a home in there, OK?"

Twenty minutes later, we walk down the hallway hand-in-hand, elated.

"I can't believe I might be pregnant at this very moment," I tell Jamie, who smiles and hugs me into him. But soon, shouts near the nurses' station prick our bubble of bliss. A man yells that his wife had two embryos transferred when they only agreed to have one transferred.

"We didn't want two," he yells with a thick accent. "She can't carry two." He gestures toward his wife who's sitting in a chair, crying. She's petite, about my size.

If she can't carry both, I think, *then neither can I.*

Suddenly, I'm terrified. Now that the embryos are inside my womb, the prospect of twins terrifies me.

Even though the head nurse points to the paperwork where the non-English-speaking wife signed off on two embryos, the husband insists that they only wanted one. But the damage is already done. I imagine all the repercussion caused by this one tiny miscommunication. Lately I've come to terms with the fact that everyone makes mistakes, but I think about this couple, and how a mistake could mean an extra, unwanted human life. And what about the other enormous IVF errors that have flashed through my newsfeed, like doctors transferring another couple's embryos into the wrong woman?

I secretly wonder if there's some alien being inside of me and pray that the embryos just implanted into my uterus belong to us, that there were, in fact, only two of them, as shown in our picture, and that the thawing didn't hinder their development.

Chapter

19

I expect to feel the weight of two marbles in my abdomen, but I feel completely, undoubtedly, the same. What *has* grown inside my uterus and attached to my insides, however, is the anxiety that I am killing our babies. Among the toxic culprits are the unrecognizable ingredients in my breakfast bars and my acne-fighting face creams that will surely zap our two embryos like zits.

I splurge and surround myself with organic, chemical-free, peace-inducing produce and products and publications. I listen to *You: Having a Baby* CDs and read pregnancy books and take prenatal vitamins and go to bed early and do visualization exercises. I know that I am going a bit overboard, but now that we were finally able to transfer the embryos, I don't want to take any risks.

Since I am used to jogging and doing yoga, the nurse's warning to "take it easy" stumps me. Can I jog, but just lightly? What does "take it easy" mean, exactly? Last October, the doctors said the same thing, and look how that turned out. I don't want to do anything that will harm our embryos. I'm afraid, even, to stand up too quickly in class. I have no idea how gentle to be with myself. Every movement feels like it might put our babies in jeopardy, yet movement is the only thing that calms my brain.

So, I walk—on the track by our house and up and down the hilly neighborhoods near my campus. But what if I get overheated and my core temperature escalates, making for a less-than-ideal environment in my womb? What if my pace is too fast and the embryos bounce around too intensely? What if my heavy breathing restricts oxygen to my uterus? What if a baseball from the neighboring athletic field sails over and socks me right in the stomach? With these fears in mind, I do a sort of stiff, non-jostling, exaggerated-breath, gimp-walk.

Are all IVF women OCD like this? I wonder. *Is this what the conception quest does to us? Makes us worry that we will lose the lives inside of us if we breathe too hard?*

The lack of the social satisfaction that I used to get from my exercise classes and the fact that, again, we're not telling anyone for fear of jinxing—these things leave me feeling so utterly lonely. I have to cancel wine nights with Kelly. I'm exhausted and impatient while teaching. Even though my heart craves companionship, I also secretly wish my Chicago friend, Marie, weren't coming to visit. I was elated when she bought her ticket a month ago, hoping I could offer her distraction, support, as it will be near the anniversary of her mom's death. But now I realize she'll be here when we get our pregnancy test results. If they are negative, I fear that I'm going to be the one who needs consoling, when I should be comforting her.

The one thing that cheers me up, is that at night, Jamie and I lie on our L-shaped sectional and talk to my stomach. I lift my shirt and roll down my pajama pants while he places his hand on the area we imagine my uterus to be. I hope that the more we pretend like something is developing inside of me, the more it will be true.

I'm having cravings that are, for sure, pregnancy related. Chicken skin and chocolate milk are my vices of choice—this from a health-conscious woman with lactose issues.

As I skin my second rotisserie chicken in the parking lot of Shaw's before I even make it home, I repeat the mantra, *I must be pregnant, I must be pregnant, I must be pregnant.* Because, otherwise, I've got serious issues.

But what about the crap they're injecting in this bird and what about the caffeine in the cocoa syrup of my chocolate milk? By this point, I can't care anymore. Worrying is exhausting. So, I just give in and peel another glistening layer of slimy, herby skin off of the steaming rotisserie chicken in my passenger seat.

I'm also making the same choices that an expectant mother would. I say no to caffeine and alcohol. My friend Jenny's mom passes away, and I want to fly to Chicago to comfort her, but the change in altitude poses a risk of miscarriage, so I have to stay put in Massachusetts.

I want to fast-forward time.

How do we go about our normal routines—work, dinner, sleep—when it feels like we should be designing a nursery and researching obstetricians?

My brain goes back and forth between convincing myself that I am pregnant and convincing myself that I am not. Jamie and I don't know whether it's OK to feel optimistic. One day we talk about the pregnancy as if we've already found out the good news. Other days we talk in conditionals. We say that we shouldn't get too invested, but we were invested the second we saw our embryos on the screen during our transfer. Every night, Jamie stares at the embryo picture on our fridge and examines their ball of cells. I wonder if he, like me, looks for faces and limbs among their circles. Sometimes, I stare at our embryos so long I expect them to climb out of the photo paper and onto my palm.

There is a pregnancy test that beckons me from the medicine cabinet like a bottle of bourbon calls out to an alcoholic. But the doctor warned us against taking home tests. I wonder, *What level of HCG does my test recognize? If it gives me a positive sign for even a low level, could it be a sign that the embryos did attach, but never developed? And would the progesterone I'm taking give me a false positive? If I take the test too early, will I cause myself unnecessary disappointment? If I take the test, and it's positive, will I jinx it and not have a positive blood test next week? Am I crazy for believing in jinxing? Am I even more insane for wearing my same "In the midst of difficulty lies opportunity" necklace every day as my good luck charm?*

Yes.

I know the answer is yes.

I have always been a little anxious, but IVF has made me full-blown crazy.

Finally, I crack.

Five days after the transfer, a week before my period is due, I ransack the medicine cabinet for the test. Because HCG levels double each day from the moment of implantation, at this point, there might be a trace of HCG detectable in my urine. So, with a shaky hand, I tear open the plastic wrapper and take the test, then place it on the counter.

I try to listen for Jamie's truck turning into our driveway but only hear the chirping birds. Just to be sure, I lock the bathroom door. If he catches me, he'll wonder why I haven't listened to the doctor, why I'm voluntarily messing with my own emotions. And I won't have a good answer for him.

My racing pulse pounds in my ears. I try to look at the bathroom curtain but keep glancing at the test on the counter where the ink lines are starting to form.

What will I do if the test is negative?

What will I do if it's positive?

There's a sudden noise outside, and my breathing halts, but when it gets closer, I realize it's the neighbor's lawn mower.

I look back at the counter.

Two dark-blue vertical lines spread across the test window.

It is surreal. If the lines appeared that quickly, then there must be a lot of HCG in my body. Surely a baby is developing inside of me. Since Tessa is the only one around, I kneel down and nuzzle into her fur, kissing her a gazillion times.

"Finally," I say out loud, wiping the creases of my eyes. "Finally."

Just five minutes after the two vertical lines appear, I head upstairs to get the Vitello bib out of my drawer so I can announce the news to Jamie when he gets home. It's then that I have a sinking realization. When I bought the test last month, I threw out the test box and directions. The stick had just been sitting in its lonely package on the top shelf of our medicine cabinet. Usually two lines means pregnant, one means not, but what were the special symbols for this brand of test?

I hop in the car and speed to CVS, still hopeful, but nervous that someone we know will be there and find me looking at the pregnancy tests.

An elderly woman has parked her cart and cane right in front of the family planning section and is looking at adult diapers on the other side of the aisle. It takes all of my strength not to climb over her.

Coughing, shaking my keys—nothing gets her attention. I

make a fake call on my cell phone so she'll hear my voice. Still nothing. Finally, she rolls her squeaky cart away. I search the boxes for the stick that looks like mine, and see right there, right on the front of the box, that two vertical lines means *not* pregnant, whereas a vertical line and a plus-sign means pregnant.

The blood drains from my face and rushes to the hives on my chest. I want to grab the test boxes and hurl them at the wall. And after that, I'll head over to the canisters of baby formula, the tubes of diaper cream, and I'll throw those, too. I want to look up and scream at the universe: *Enough. We've paid our dues. We've put in our time. We deserve some good news. Please, for the love of God, stop fucking with us.*

But there is one consolation that I find on the back of the box in my hands. The directions say that the earliest you should take the test is four days before your missed period, which would be three days from now. I've taken the test too early.

I still might have a reason to pull out our Vitello bib, after all.

With a new box of pregnancy tests, I emerge from the store into the sunny afternoon, and tell myself that I can take one every morning for the next three days, just in case a bit of HCG miraculously shows up.

When I get home, operation hide-the-pregnancy-tests begins. If Jamie sees them, he'll side with the doctor about waiting until the official blood test, and I don't think I could honestly promise him that. In a process that's beyond my control, the tests are the one thing that can offer answers.

In the morning, upon exiting the shower, something strikes me in the mirror—my breasts. They are bigger, as are my areolas, which have more braille bumps. And I'm not even imagining this. Jamie agrees and stares at them as he brushes his teeth.

I towel off, glancing anxiously at my pregnancy test hiding

spot, hoping he won't move the face cloths and find the wands. "This wait is killing me," I tell him. In our cramped bathroom, we sidestep each other as he spits out his toothpaste and I apply deodorant. "I just want to know. Don't you?"

He rinses his toothbrush and says, "I'm just trying not to think about it."

He's been working more lately, checking his work email more at night. I just thought he had extra projects, but this must be his way of staying occupied. I look at the medicine cabinet again, knowing that, instead of working late or checking email, I'll be racing home tonight to take another test.

Two days before our official pregnancy test, the night before Marie flies in, I awake to strong period cramps and a horrendous backache, worse than any I've ever had. Jamie and Tessa snore away next to me. The house is still and dark. The warm night air wafts in through the open window. It seems that the rest of the world is at peace, but I am not. My back muscles clench in pain, and my pajama pants are going to be full of blood, I just know it.

This is it.

This is the end.

One monster fear consumes me—*What if I see the embryos in the blood? What if they already look like miniature babies, and when I wipe, I can see their little bodies?*

If that happens, I'll die.

My thumping heart and racing feet get me downstairs in five seconds flat. I sprint past the picture of the embryos on our fridge, but I don't dare look at them.

On instinct, I flick the bathroom light on and my pupils shrink. Then I flick the switch back off, not wanting to see the evidence in my underwear.

I pull my pants down, sit on the toilet.

There is going to be so much blood.

When I wipe, I can't see anything in the dark, so I hold the light switch between my fingers and slowly flick it on.

Inhale.

Exhale.

I look down at the toilet paper, then at my pants, expecting red paper and red fabric.

But there's nothing, just the white toilet paper and my white underwear.

I wipe myself again.

Still nothing.

I can't believe there's nothing.

The embryos are still inside of me.

Thank you, I whisper to whatever higher power is guiding this world.

Thank you.

Chapter

20

On the morning of the blood pregnancy test, I pull our wrinkled Vitello bib out of my drawer and fold it into my pocket. The nurse is scheduled to call in the early afternoon. I have the day off, but Jamie is working. So, the plan is that Jamie will take his lunch and meet Marie and me at a restaurant. When the nurse calls, Jamie and I will step out to answer the call. I'll put the nurse on speakerphone and we'll get the good news. I'll pull out the bib so that we can look at it, reflect on our long journey, and rejoice that we can finally make use of the garment. We can walk back inside the restaurant and tell Marie that I'm pregnant.

It's a bright August day, and Marie squints to look for spots as I circle the Patriot's Place parking lot. Patriot's Place is the retail center that borders the football stadium, and I picked it because it's close to Jamie's work and has plenty of restaurant options. People in jerseys swarm the lot, and it's then that I realize that today is the first preseason game. As fans shout and cheer, I hope that we, too, will have something to celebrate.

At Skip Jack's, I can't even concentrate on anything that the waitress is saying because I keep staring at my phone, willing the nurse to call. The waitress brings us water, and my phone doesn't ring. She takes our order, and still, it doesn't ring. Marie chats with us, and I want so badly to carry on a conversation with her, but I can't process any kind of normal response. Despite the AC, Jamie's sweat rolls from his hairline to the collar of his work shirt.

When my phone vibrates in my hand, I jump up, almost knocking over my water glass.

Jamie and I emerge from the restaurant and are stifled by the heat. My heart pounds as we walk out onto the promenade near the football stadium. I hoped there would be some private place where we could talk, but Patriots fans are everywhere. It's a sea of blue and red and I have to shout over their cheers to answer the phone.

But as soon as the nurse says hello, I know.

"It's not good," I mouth to Jamie. And it isn't.

"I'm so sorry," the nurse says.

I drop to the cement and press my face into my knees. Jamie squats down next to me, his cheeks growing redder by the second.

A minute later our doctor calls us.

"If I'm not pregnant, why haven't I gotten my period?" I grill him, as if this will change the results of my pregnancy test.

He explains that the progesterone I've been taking is the reason for my enlarged chest and my lack of a menstrual cycle.

He says we can try again, but I'm not hearing any of it.

"I am so done with IVF," I shout, and I hang up the phone.

Jamie tries to hug and kiss me. He kneels down next to me in his work pants and blocks the crowd with his body so that they won't stare at his hysterical wife having a meltdown in front of a stadium where everyone else is happy and tipsy.

I always thought that if a husband and wife suffered a common loss, it'd be slightly easier to endure because they could comfort each other. But I was wrong. So terribly wrong. I knew nothing of shared sorrow. Until now.

Because Jamie isn't crying, and because I want to put my pain on a platter and present it to someone else, I take the Vitello bib from my pocket and throw it into his lap. "I guess we won't be needing this," I say.

I don't squeeze his hand and say it will be OK. I hurl that bib at Jamie like it is all his fault.

How morbidly ironic it is that we never acknowledged the full meaning of Vitello, of veal. It isn't just baby cow, it's *dead* baby cow.

I charge away from the restaurant, through the throngs of jerseys and shopping bags, to my car, abandoning Marie in the restaurant, leaving Jamie to box our food and pay our bill. Angry energy pulses in my toes. I could sprint the thirty miles back to our home, I'm sure of it. Caveman adrenaline courses through my arteries, daring me to outsprint the negative news that's chasing me.

Marie and I had planned to kayak that afternoon, and when Jamie finds me crying in the parking lot, he suggests that we still go. It will be good for me, he says. I don't fight him or insist that he and I be together so that he can comfort me or I can comfort him. Instead, he gets into his truck, and Marie and I get into my car.

I can't believe that I have to suck up my sadness and spend my afternoon entertaining someone, I think. But, luckily, Marie doesn't expect to be entertained. As we drive to Hopkinton State Park, she says that we could just sit in silence, whatever I want.

I ramble.

She listens.

I cry until snot fills my nose. When we park, she leans over the center console and hugs me. Marie is a social worker by trade and knows just how to handle my raging anger. Be-

cause of losing her mom unexpectedly last year, she understands loss far beyond what I've just experienced. She's had
enough people try to console her in the worst ways, so she
knows exactly what not to say. She tells me how, soon after
her mother died, someone tried to empathize by sharing the
story of their dog's death. The pure stupidity of people actually
makes us laugh. I am so glad she's here. She's exactly the friend
I need right now.

We row around Hopkinton's lake and talk. As we churn
the oars, sweat and sadness pour out of us.

Afterward, as Marie rests in the sun, I swim, yearning to
flutter-kick the sadness and the dead embryos out of me. I
want no reminders that we lost two balls of cells that felt like
our babies. When Marie and I get back into my car and head
home, I contemplate throwing my *You: Having a Baby* CDs on
the pavement and running them over.

The next day, after dropping Marie off at the airport, I
sprint up hills until the walls of my lungs stretch thin.

Over the next week, I drink wine and caffeine and eat
sushi and do hot yoga and get my hair highlighted. Fill me up
on chemicals and stimulants and downers and endorphins. I
am going to fly at the highest altitudes and do all the things
that pregnancy forbade. From now on, I am going to be selfish.

Day after day, I slither out of Jamie's grasp. I shoot him
evil looks. I am mad that IVF didn't take over his life for the
past year as it did mine. I detest him for not having a scar on
his abdomen or mood swings from synthetic hormones. Because I can't yell at the embryos or the reproductive specialists
or at my own body for failing me, I build a slanderous cam-
paign against the one person I love most.

Unlike me, I argue internally, Jamie didn't have to leave
the house an hour early every morning to go for ultrasounds
and blood work and get bad technicians who stabbed and col-

lapsed his veins. He wasn't required to wait by the phone between two and five each afternoon hoping the day's results would warrant moving on to the next step. He wasn't mentally absent from his job.

The rift between us widens.

I loathe his inability to elaborate on his feelings.

"I'm angry. I'm sad," he says. "What else do you want me to say?"

The more I rant about my despair and rage, the more Jamie recoils.

One day, I'm hanging clothes in my closet and Jamie's standing in the doorway, when I tell him I wish that he had gone through all of the hard stuff—the testing and procedures—instead of me. I tell him I can't imagine our future without kids.

"Maybe you need a partner who can give you children naturally," he says without emotion.

I cock my head, wondering if I heard him right. Because what I heard was this: *I am not the right person for you and I don't want to be the right person for you.* I heard: *Maybe you made the wrong decision marrying me. Maybe I made the wrong decision marrying you. Maybe we never should have married each other. Maybe we shouldn't be married right now. Maybe we should get divorced.*

Because even though I told him that I can't imagine a future without a baby, I still can't imagine a future without Jamie. I hate him so much in that moment for suggesting I need a new partner that I want to hit him with the hanger in my hand.

I leave the clothes in a heap on the bed, and sprint out of the house for a run, pushing my legs to move at the same sprinting speed of my mind. I ask myself, *What if he's right? What if we made a mistake in marrying each other?* I imagine my new life, sans Jamie. *I'll be single and free of this IVF mess,* I think, *and I'll . . . I'll . . . What?* Every ending to that sentence feels so empty. So I'll have more free time. And I'll busy myself with writing or some other hobby. And then what? I'll find myself searching the earth for the same partner that I already have right in front of me.

That night, I drink red wine and fling the Polaroid of our embryo-flowers onto our bedroom floor along with my pregnancy handbook. Jamie is downstairs in front of the TV, repulsed by my seething. I am upstairs, repulsed by the obnoxious volume of his movie viewing. He's watching some war film, and the rapid fire shooting sounds as if someone has opened up an automatic rifle in our own living room.

I look around our bedroom at the pictures from six years ago, when we first met. I cry and cry thinking about how giddy we used to be. I remember who I was then, who Jamie made me into—a person capable of love. I think of how I always held his hand and how weeks apart felt like an eternity and how I bunny-hopped down the aisle the day we got married and how badly I wanted to have his babies. Our marriage doesn't feel like it was a mistake.

The next morning, I awake, and the embryo flower photo is sitting on Jamie's dresser. The Vitello bib rests on his nightstand.

How can he stand the evidence of what we don't have? I wonder.

I tell everyone I know about our loss. He tells no one. He goes into work on a Saturday even though he doesn't need to. I go to Barnes & Noble, flip through magazines, listen to sad music on my laptop, email friends about our pseudo-miscarriage. I ask them to say that they are here for us and are sorry for our loss. I cry in public at all the babies and toddlers that stroll past the window.

With every condolence email that friends send, I feel more supported, less alone.

As a truce, before exiting the strip mall, I call Jamie to see what he wants for dinner. There's so much tension between us that our voices are both strained and the conversation is awkward. He asks, sarcastically, for a lobster roll and chocolate lava cake because we live in the boonies and neither of these things are readily available, but then he says, seriously, that he wants nothing.

Quickly, my frustration with him grows. "You have to eat something," I say, but he insists he's not hungry.

I want him to say he's been crying, publicly, like I have. Instead, he says it's been crazy at work. My molars grind together.

Why hasn't he spent his hours thinking about our babies instead of business? I want to know.

While walking to my car, I get a text from Marie.

She says she loves me and is thinking of me.

It's such a simple thing, but so profound. I pause in the sidewalk to read it again. People with shopping bags bump into me, but I stand there rereading it and realize this: I never said these very words to my own husband. I sent an email asking my family and friends for support, yet I haven't given Jamie the very thing I asked other people for. Since learning of the pregnancy results, I haven't once said, "I love you" or "I am here for you."

If a friend can say these things to me, why can't I say these same words to my husband? Why can't I ignore his hard exterior and understand that he went to work on a Saturday because he's hurting? That he isn't eating because nothing can fill the void of the lives we lost? What if he said that I should have a different spouse because he's blaming himself for us not having children? What if he stayed downstairs blasting movies last night because he thought I was upstairs plotting our separation?

If Jamie were my friend instead of my husband, I think, if I had not lost the babies, too, how would I be treating him right now?

Remembering that during the summer in New England, Panera offers lobster rolls, I head there and buy Jamie one along with a fudge brownie. It's not a chocolate lava cake, but, hopefully, it will do. On my drive home, I vow to comfort Jamie and to disregard my own pain for the evening. I will use my sorrow to try and understand his. Every time he feigns indifference, I'll caress him. I am going to give him everything that I asked my family and friends for in my earlier email—a listening ear, words of love. I am going to treat him as if the loss is separate from me. Tonight, the loss is not ours, not mine, but his. When I come home, I set out our dinner with a flourish. Even still, Jamie won't eat. Though my heart hardens a little, I put the food in the fridge and sit down on the living room floor where he's lounging with Tessa. My fingers stroke his scalp. I don't ask him to talk. We move onto the couch, and I rub his head some more. Every time I kiss the dog, I kiss Jamie, too. Eventually, Jamie eats the lobster roll and the brownie.

In a small voice, he says, "Thank you."

Later, when he falls asleep in bed, I continue to massage his head. My arms and legs entwine his. Even in his slumber, I hold him. And it makes me want to cry less—channeling my energy not into running or throwing, but into caressing my husband.

The next morning, in return, before we get out of bed, Jamie wraps his arm around me. He combs my hair with his fingers. He kisses my neck.

The bib still sits on his nightstand. We are still without child.

But we *have* conceived something after all of this—the ability to comfort each other through loss.

Of the long, winding trip we've been on, this is our souvenir.

PART III

Chapter

21

Today is the eleventh anniversary of September eleventh. Jamie dresses for work, and I wake up slowly as the radio murmurs. The station he listens to while getting ready usually plays classic rock, but today, patriotic tributes interrupt the songs.

Jamie kisses me goodbye, and I lie in bed for a little longer than usual. Since I teach four weekdays and all day on Saturday, Tuesdays are my day off. I cherish these peaceful mornings and usually lounge in bed a little while after Jamie leaves. It gives me the rare opportunity to actually sit and reflect. And I do so now as I listen to the radio.

Everyone who calls into the station seems upbeat, telling only tales of courage—how, because of the September 11th terror, we came together as a nation and emerged victorious.

I wonder how the people of New York feel about the idea of balance. Do they think that because they experienced such terror, good fortune will come in equal measures? Or do they think that balance is a lie that people recite so that they don't go mad with rage?

Nowadays, Jamie and I ponder the notion of balance and karma. Jamie will list the misfortunes he's already experienced, like his cancer and the fire that took his possessions just two years after that. He'll say, "I must have been an asshole in some other life."

And I, ever the optimist, usually say fortune-cookie things, like, "Life balances out. Good things are bound to come our way."

In yoga, I once heard a quote comparing life to an arrow. "An arrow can only be shot by pulling it backward," the instructor read aloud, "so when life is dragging you back with difficulties, that means it's going to launch you into something great."

Despite its cheesiness, I loved the quote, until I noticed that life was doing a whole lot of pulling and not nearly enough launching. As of late, I've been uttering my affirmations less and less, because, the truth is, I don't believe them anymore. That higher power that's supposed to even out the scales, the one I've always believed balanced the bad with the good—I'm not so sure it exists anymore. Otherwise, I wouldn't have almost bled to death or lost our two transferred embryos. If balance existed, we'd have a baby in our arms.

But we don't.

After the failed transfer last month, I declared that I was done with IVF, and we went on vacation to forget about it all, but just a couple of days ago, Dr. Peters ran more tests and said that it was unlikely we'd ever get pregnant naturally.

Now here we are again, with no baby and no options.

I shut off the radio and head downstairs to the bathroom. As I'm about to undress for the shower, I look for razors in the vanity cabinet and notice my box of unused tampons. When I pull my shorts down, I find my underwear unspotted and realize that my period never came last night.

I'm late.

The sun shines through the bathroom, and I think, *Imagine*

if I found out today, of all days, that I was pregnant naturally. Imagine if the sex marathon that Jamie and I had two weeks ago actually did the trick. Was that really all it took? Some relaxation in New Hampshire and spontaneous sex?

My pregnancy tests beckon me from their hidden spot in the medicine cabinet behind my face wash.

Just undress and get in the shower, I order myself. *This is ridiculous. The doctor said that it was impossible.*

But even with my socks and shorts stripped off, I'm still thinking about the tests. Through the wood of the cabinet, my x-ray vision spots them.

Maybe just one, says my heart.

To which my brain fumes: *Really? You're going to do this to yourself again?*

On its own accord, my arm reaches out. My hand opens the door, rifling through soaps and towels until it finds my hiding spot. My fingers grab the box, which advertises two lines on a test and the word "pregnant" in large font above the wand.

I pee on the stick without regard for aim or positioning and set it on the sink, not looking at it, so deep is my shame.

My wiser self approaches the podium for a lecture.

Why do you will these tests to lie to you? How many sticks have you purchased in the last year and a half? And haven't they all come out negative? How many hours of false hope and disappointment have these damn tests caused you? Why, oh, why, do you keep doing this to yourself?

To the garbage I am about to send the stick. But then, two lines peer back at me.

A positive test.

Is it possible?

Can this really be?

Then doubt steals my hope.

Did I look at the package too quickly? What if, like last time, this is one of the tests that's supposed to have a plus sign?

But, right there, in bold print on the box, it says that two vertical lines means pregnant. It's not convincing enough. I need to take another one. I want to shower fast and guzzle water so that I'll pee right away, but I force myself to lather up slowly. If my urine is too weak, the test won't pick up the HCG hormone.

As the steaming water massages my skin, I pretend that this is a normal shower, though, of course, my thoughts are already time-traveling through the next nine months.

My loofah knows the drill—left shoulder, bicep, forearm, fingers, palm, then reverse, armpits, chest, neck, right shoulder, bicep, forearm, fingers, palm, reverse, ribs, stomach, back, butt, thighs, hamstrings, shins, calves, ankles, soles, toes, reverse. I shampoo my scalp, rinse my hair, put conditioner on my ponytail, leave it there while I exfoliate my face, shave my armpits, bikini line, legs, rinse my conditioner, then turn off the water.

I pull back the shower curtain and look toward the sink. The stick still shows the dark lines. Then, dripping wet, I take a new test.

It's instantly positive.

Shaking, I take a picture of the tests with my phone as irrefutable evidence for the naysayers in my mind.

A smile spreads across my face, but my skepticism quickly wipes it away. Because of my previous false hope after the embryo transfer when I saw two vertical lines, I don't even believe the results. These two tests don't seem definitive enough. A digital one that reads either "pregnant" or "not pregnant" is the only thing that will stop my second-guessing.

I'm in the car driving to CVS before I even notice my mismatched shorts and tank top. Houses on both sides of the street fly American flags.

When I walk through the pharmacy's sliding automatic

doors, a voice—a new voice, a nurturing voice—says *Remember this*, because unlike every other time I've entered this store, right now, I could be entering the store as a truly, undeniably pregnant person.

This time, when I buy the box, I do not cower with shame and look at the magazines. I look the cashier in the eye and smile. Though I want to speed home, again that voice whispers: *Slow down, you might be carrying precious cargo.*

At home, Tessa follows me into the bathroom. She's wagging her tail, feeding off of my endorphins. I leave the door open and unwrap the package slowly, then pee on precisely the spot drawn in the directions. Unlike all the other times I've taken a test, once the stick is percolating on the bathroom sink, I walk away. The stove clock says 8:25, and I unload the dishwasher, forcing myself to wait until 8:27. My eyes never leave the glowing clock numbers. Plates clatter as I stack them in the cabinet next to the stove, and it seems that the clock is broken. It remains on 8:26 for an eternity. Then, finally, the six morphs into a seven. I take a deep breath and consider one last possibility. What if life is like one giant store, and the larger the purchase you make, the more you pay for it with sacrifice? What if all the things we've been through were a down payment for the price of a baby?

I walk back to the bathroom with forced slowness, preparing myself to see the "not" of the "not pregnant."

I open the door and tiptoe to the stick.

My eyes look for the "not" and look for the "not" and look for the "not," but it's not there.

The only thing it says is "pregnant."

I cry-laugh and jump up and down and hug Tessa and cry-laugh some more.

So, if I am pregnant, I think, *does that mean that this baby is a miracle or that the doctors were wrong?*

A couple of days ago, when Dr. Peters said it was improbable for us to get pregnant without IVF, the cells of our naturally conceived embryo were multiplying. As he explained that our vacation Jacuzzi soaks and Jamie's brief-style underwear further diminished our nonexistent chances, I was pregnant.

Just as when we'd been told that Jamie's sperm analysis from last October was better, there's the question I can't contemplate for more than a second because it sours my stomach: *Could we have avoided almost two years of heartache if we hadn't been sold a completely unnecessary procedure? Would we have saved ourselves physical pain and marital strain if we'd have been just a little more patient and not run to the doctors for help?*

But we'd been told again and again that we couldn't conceive naturally. Now, I punish myself: *I shouldn't have trusted them. I should have gotten a third opinion. I should have read more books. I should have . . . I should have . . .*

I have to shake my head to stop the continuous ring of regrets.

When I go to Jamie's office and reveal the news, he's just as ecstatic and shocked as I am. He stares at my stomach and shakes his head, saying, "They told us it couldn't happen . . ."

"I know," I say, grinning, "but it did."

"I can't believe it," he says, his eyes glistening. He hugs me hard and then pulls back, afraid he's harming the baby somehow.

"It's OK," I say, laughing, and he hugs me again.

Now, we must wait some more—for me to get my blood drawn, for the lab to call at the end of the day with the results.

After work, Jamie meets me at Panera, and we await the nurse's call. We want to drive to Jamie's parents' house and announce the news if it's positive, and they live just ten minutes from here. Our house is a twenty-minute drive in the opposite direction, and the nurse is due to ring us any minute now, so it makes sense just to stay here, but a fear festers. *What if this call is like the last one?* This might very well be the second time we hear horrific news in public and the second time I collapse on a sidewalk in front of strangers.

We step outside into the warm afternoon and stand on the sidewalk with nowhere to go. I stare out at the parking lot, the gas station, and the street beyond that, as if we're standing before some beautiful beach, watching the waves crash.

Finally, my phone rings, startling us. I put it on speakerphone so we can both listen. This means that other strip-mall shoppers will hear the news, too. But if the results are positive, nothing else will matter.

My heart pounds and I think of the arrow quote. I can feel the universe gripping us in its mighty hand. *Please,* I think, *please launch us. Please don't pull us back.*

The nurse says that, shockingly, these things do happen from time to time. Her voice sounds happy, but what does she mean by "these things"—natural pregnancy after IVF or false positives on home pregnancy tests?

"Your HCG was 62," she says.

"That's good, right?" I ask. "You wanted it above 50?"

"That's right."

Jamie and I mouth "Oh my God" to each other as we struggle to stay focused and listen.

The nurse congratulates us and adds that I have to return for blood work on Thursday to assure that the levels have doubled, but that everything looks good right now. We can get an ultrasound in three weeks to hear the heartbeat.

It seems absolutely impossible that there is a human being growing inside my body who is growing a heart inside its own body.

We hang up, and Jamie and I stare at each other for a good long second, in awe.

Though a million fears like miscarriage and a C-section delivery beat at the walls of my mind, I try to enjoy this and not let it be clouded by the worry that has followed us for so long.

Chapter

22

"Have you been smoking weed?" Jamie asks, laughing. "You're so chill."

He's right. I am, for the first time in my life, all sorts of Zen. Our baby is channeling my inner Buddha. It's as if someone has slowed down time. I feel no urge to rush or tackle my to-do list. It feels like I've had a nice big glass of wine.

Other pregnancy perks include thicker hair and a fuller chest. I have not a single complaint about being with child. Which makes me wonder, *What are all those women on Baby Center whining about?*

Morning sickness, wacky cravings, hemorrhoids, mood swings—I've escaped them all, and I cuddle on Jamie's lap, content. The last two weeks have been nothing but blissful. My second set of HCG results were 211—well above the 124 the doctor had hoped for—proof that our baby's cells are multiplying healthily.

We finally get to announce the news we've been waiting to share for almost two years.

"How do you feel about being a grandmother?" I ask when I call Mom up at work. She cheers so loudly that I have to hold the phone away from my ear.

When I ring Dana, she repeats, "Oh my God. I can't believe it. Oh my God," about thirty times.

But I most love watching Jamie tell his parents. I've never seen Jamie look so proud. We sit at George and Judi's kitchen table. Jamie shows them pictures of our vacation in New Hampshire, casually describing the cabin and the nearby pond. "And then," he adds, "when we came back, Nadine got pregnant."

George and Judi both tilt their heads, confused. Then they see the giant smile on Jamie's face, and they start laughing and crying.

But my favorite part is that Jamie and I are "us" again. We are the couple we used to be before IVF took over our lives. I write Jamie love notes and snuggle in the recliner with him after dinner. Before bed, I massage his scalp. We steal smooches every chance we get. When we stand in line at the grocery store, Jamie places his hand on my back. I send him spontaneous texts to tell him I'm thinking of him. We look at each other as if no other being exists in the universe. And I love seeing Jamie look happy again. He sings for no reason. He drums the steering wheel when he drives. He tells jokes. He plays with the dog. God, how I've missed him. I had no idea what the IVF process had stolen from us until we got it back.

Today, we have our ultrasound at the fertility clinic. If the pregnancy is viable, we'll be released to a normal obstetrician, which means we'll never have to step foot in the depressing clinic again. If the pregnancy isn't viable, well then . . . I can't even bring myself to think about that.

I dress in leggings, a tank top, and a light cardigan. The thin clothes serve two functions: 1. to keep me cool now that I'm always hot, and 2. to show off the teeny-tiny roundness that I am calling my bump. Yes, I'm one of those annoying

pregnant women who's going to flaunt this baby every chance
I get. It's not as much about showing off the miracle of life as it
is displaying the reward for all of our sacrifice. It's a way of
proving that despite all of the tests and appointments, all of the
injections and failures, we triumphed.

Jamie and I drive to the clinic talking positively. We say
that we're convinced this is the real deal. But, inside, nervousness paralyzes my body and brain. We park and unbuckle, but
I'm not quite sure I can get my leaden legs to step out of the
truck.

Jamie walks over to my side and holds out his hand.

Unlike all of our other visits, we are ushered to a part of
the building I didn't even know existed—the secret section
where the happy people go. I wonder if the ultrasound room is
purposely stationed separately so that people who receive sad
news don't have to see the gloating faces of those who get to
view their long-awaited babies on a screen.

Even the ultrasound technician is shockingly bubbly. After
I get into position on the padded table, she hands me an ultrasound wand and says, in a singsongy voice, "OK, if you'll just
insert that, in a minute here, we'll see your uterus, then your
baby, then the heart." Opposite of all our other experiences at
the clinic, where we were spoken to in conditionals, now,
there are no "ifs" or "maybes" recited to us. It's been a long time
since we've heard "you will" instead of "you might."

The next minute of breath holding while she manipulates
the wand and taps on her keyboard is torture. The stampede of
worry I was unable to process on the drive now charges
through my mind. *What if my uterus is empty? What if there's a
fetus but no heartbeat?*

In the dark room, Jamie and I stare at the small gray
screen, awaiting the news that will either thrill us or crush us.
Jamie, as always, hides his apprehension and pats my arm, as if

to say, "Here we go." I think about the other times he has been in this position—standing over my body on a medical table. Each time, he has somehow swallowed his own fear, gripped my hand, and extracted all of my anxiety through his fingertips, then taken it into his own body and stored it away in the deep pockets of his organs.

In silent gratitude, I rub his hand, tracing the Celtic knots on his wedding ring.

The technician moves the wand and clicks the zoom button until the monitor displays what looks like an oval lake and a little white peninsula at the bottom. "This," she says, tracing the oval on the screen, "is your uterus. This," she says, pointing to the lake, "is your amniotic fluid. And this," she says, zooming in on the peninsula, "is your baby."

Jamie and I simultaneously lean forward, squint, and shake our heads.

With its block-shaped head and nubby arms, our baby looks like the most beautiful miniature T. rex I've ever seen.

Jamie kisses my hand over and over again.

I want to jump up and cheer, but we still don't know if there's a heartbeat. Unbeknownst to me, the baby could have stopped developing. It's the size of a lentil, and I certainly can't feel it yet, so how can I be positive that it's alive?

I think of how happy Jamie and I are, and how quickly that can go away if we find out there's no heartbeat.

Please, please, please, I chant. *Please give us this gift.*

Then, the tech zooms in even more. She points her cursor to two vertical flickering lines and says, "And this is your baby's heart."

After measuring the beats per minute, she plays the galloping heartbeat for us.

How can I explain the joy of hearing rapid, steady hooves running along the field of my eardrums?

I'm speechless.

"We're looking for at least 120 beats per minute," she says, "and we've got 133 here. That's great."

Jamie smiles bigger than I've ever seen him smile and leans down to kiss me.

This is foreign to us—receiving good news without footnotes of "until the next test" or "for now." We don't even know how to react. We stare at the screen, then at each other, then back to the screen, and shake our heads.

The tech measures the baby, proclaiming it six weeks and five days old. "Your due date is May 19," she says.

I want to jump up on the table and shout, "We're going to have a BABY!!!" at the top of my lungs, but the tech still has to check my cervix.

Because I've had two LEEP procedures to remove abnormal cells from my cervix, I'll have to be monitored more closely than most women. The good thing is that this means plenty of ultrasounds and glimpses at the baby, whereas most women only get two ultrasounds per pregnancy. But the bad news is that, because of the LEEP procedures, my cervix might be thin. Thin isn't good because the cervix is like the plug that keeps the uterus and the baby in place. If I have too slim of a cervix, my risk of miscarriage increases.

The tech drags her cursor across a small patch of flesh on the screen and measures it. She smiles and says that it could change as the pregnancy progresses, but right now, my cervix looks good.

"Want to see something cool?" she adds as she moves the wand to focus on one of my ovaries.

She points to a dark circle. "That is your corpus luteum," she says, "which means that this is the ovary that released the egg that was fertilized."

Jamie and I stare at the screen, and say, "Crazy."

"Which ovary is it?" I ask.

"Your left," she says, then she moves on to her next task, but Jamie and I look at each other in disbelief. After being pinpricked a million times from egg-retrieval needles, after hemorrhaging, after being sutured, my little ovary-that-could still got the job done.

My palm presses down on the spot beside my left hip where I picture my ovary to be.

Thank you, I tell it. *Thank you.*

Kelly and Mikey are getting married in a few weeks, and Jamie and I are standing up in the wedding. We haven't been able to tell anyone about the baby besides our immediate family due to the make-it-through-the-first-trimester rule. But we agree to tell Mikey and Kelly so that we don't have to keep hiding our ultrasound photos and drinking non-alcoholic wine every time they come over.

I decide to tell the other bridesmaids as well. These women are the perfect audience because, after the wedding, I'll never see most of them again. So if something goes wrong, and I miscarry, I won't have to worry about repeating the sad news to them.

We're at Foxwoods Casino for Kelly's bachelorette party, and as we sit in the hotel room eating cheese and grapes, I brag about my fabulous pregnancy. I rub my barely there belly more than any pregnant woman should be allowed. I blab on and on about the ultrasound and the heartbeat.

Politely, Kelly and the other women listen. They even feign smiles.

Although she has every right to, Kelly does not shout, "The attention is supposed to be on *me,* not you. Please shut up."

Her curly-haired friend does not say, "My husband and I have been trying to have a baby for years, and I really don't feel like hearing your wonderful news. I'd prefer that you stop talking now."

And I could take cues from Melissa, the pregnant maid of honor, to just rest my hands in my lap and ask Kelly about her dress and her honeymoon.

But no, no, I just can't keep my big mouth shut.

It's not until later that it happens.

We're walking through the noisy casino, on our way to the Japanese restaurant for dinner. I'm blathering on to Melissa about how we're going to name the baby Geo for a boy or Raya for a girl. So, for now, we're calling the baby Raya-Geo.

When I finally pause for a breath, I hear sniffling behind me. I turn to see Kelly consoling her cousin—her cousin who's crying because she hasn't been able to conceive the sibling that her daughter begs for.

And that's when I realize what an insensitive bitch I've been.

Have I so quickly forgotten what it's like to be on the other side, listening to women boast about their nurseries and their newborns? Can't I remember the burning jealousy and how I wished repeatedly for other women to be a bit more aware, a bit more censored?

Quite abruptly, I stop talking. When we get to the restaurant, I am almost silent through entrées and dessert. Afterward, a headache bangs my forehead and nausea twirls my stomach. The other girls go dancing, but I have to head back to the hotel room lest I collapse from what feels like vertigo.

"It must be the salmon I ate," I tell Jamie when I call to wish him goodnight, but I secretly fear that this is my punishment for boasting. *OK*, I bargain with the universe, *I accept my penance. I definitely deserve this. But just one night, alright? Just as long as I feel better in the morning.*

Then the morning comes, and I have to tiptoe past sleeping bodies to the hotel bathroom, where I crouch and dry heave into the toilet. But, try as I might, nothing comes out. I chug water, and we eat a buffet breakfast. Despite wanting to gorge on Danishes and cheesy potatoes au gratin, I stick to fruit and eggs, but the headache and the nausea still follow me like a shadow.

In the bathroom again, I hunch over the toilet. Nothing. I never knew that there was something worse than vomiting—nausea that never goes away.

After breakfast, we walk through the quiet casino toward the hotel room. I see the bloodshot eyes and tired movements of the post-party gamblers who drag their suitcases. A twenty-something girl with dirty hair and smeared makeup looks back at me and smiles, like we're part of the same club.

The only difference, I think, is that her headache will be gone tomorrow.

But mine? Who knows.

I can now join the ranks of the complaining women on Baby Center.

Constipation, sore gums, nausea—every symptom the baby books mention, I get in heaping doses. My healthy diet goes to shit, as the only things I can stomach are fat and sugar. For breakfast one morning, I eat a Klondike Bar, then an hour later I drive to Panera and down a cheesy bacon breakfast sandwich and a hot chocolate with extra whip cream and marshmallows. Just like when I thought I was pregnant after our embryo transfer, my cravings also call for rotisserie chickens. There's nothing better than the glistening, salty skin, which I peel off in strips and dangle into my mouth as droplets of grease coat my tongue. Like before, I perform this ritual in the parking lot of Shaw's each afternoon. Because why should I wait until I get home when I can eat a whole chicken-hide while the skin is still steaming hot?

Jamie comes home from work one afternoon to find three bald chickens in the fridge and me, on the couch, skinning my fourth. Laughing, he takes a picture of me with his iPhone and calls me his little carnivore. He loves the pregnant version of me who—unlike the health-conscious, energetic me—says yes to chocolate cake and couch time.

Entering a grocery store these days feels like perusing the markets in Guatemala. I don't know what I'll want, so I let my nose lead the way. Just because I liked something yesterday or five minutes ago, doesn't guarantee I'll like it now. We used to shop the perimeter of the store—fruit, veggies, deli, fish, meat, eggs. Now I traverse the middle aisles, picking up things like cinnamon-dusted pumpkin seeds that I'll neglect later that evening when I deem them disgusting. And forget cooking. The smells of garlic and ground meat instantly flick my vomit switch.

Though I spent the good majority of the last eighteen months reading up on the best organic foods for a baby-in-utero, now that I'm actually pregnant, I'm eating Easy Mac for every meal. I'm chewing aspartame-ridden gum and guzzling artificially sweetened seltzer to my heart's content. Previous go-tos of apples and trail mix induce instant nausea. I drive with a sick cup in my car at all times.

Yesterday, I guzzled Nestlé chocolate milk all morning, so I tried to force in some healthy fruit on my ride home from work, only to be punished by my stomach. The light had just turned green, and braking or pulling over proved impossible, so I heaved my insides into the cup while simultaneously swerving my way home.

So, naturally, I went home to drink more chocolate milk. And though I'd normally be worried about the weighty repercussions of eating such shitty foods, the scale last night read the lowest in my adult life. Any other time, I'd rejoice at getting under the 120 mark, but now that number sends fear firing through my spinal cord. *My malnourished baby is, most definitely, doomed,* I think, *and it's all my fault.*

Sometimes, I retch my breakfast, other times I lose my lunch, but, without fail, every single night now, I throw up my dinner. Even when I think I've done alright—just eaten little bits of bland pasta, I'll sit up in bed feeling the burning clumps of bile making a pilgrimage to my mouth, and I'll have to run back downstairs. Jamie rubs my shoulders and sweeps my hair out of my face as I vomit my non-digested dinner.

I usually throw up so hard that it splashes back and hits me in the face. Sometimes I throw up and simultaneously pee my pants. Urinating myself is actually the one thing about pregnancy that humors me these days.

"I think I'm going to have to buy Depends," I tell Jamie, mustering a laugh.

Then I crawl back upstairs, prop more pillows behind me, and fall asleep in a completely upright position. My body thermostat must be off as well, because I go to bed shivering and wake up sweating. And usually, my vivid dreams disorient me so drastically that it's a good five minutes before I realize where I am in the morning.

"What's it like? Pregnancy?" my sister asks. She's in love and having the marriage-plus-babies talk with her beau.

"It's like having the worst hangover of your life every single day," I tell her as I dress for bed. It's 8:00 p.m. and even taking out my contacts feels like such a taxing chore that I contemplate leaving them in.

"You think that when you wake up in the morning, your headache will be gone, but it never goes away. You're starving, but you can't eat. And you're totally wiped out all the time. It's awesome."

"Shit, Nay," Dana says. "That sounds awful."

I used to be able to teach all day then attend nighttime writing workshops. I'd leave the house at 7:00 a.m. and return at 10:00 p.m. Nowadays, I must take each hour as it comes and say things like: *Just make it to work without puking. Just get through the first part of class until break. Just walk across campus without ralphing in public. Just get through the next class until lunchtime. Just hold down your soup and crackers. Just make it to four-thirty. Just try to exercise for a half an hour. Just make the drive home so you can rest.*

Sea bands, acupuncture, antinausea lollypops, B vitamins— nothing works.

Though I've joked with Dana and Jamie about my hangover that never goes away, it's not funny anymore. More food leaves my mouth than enters it. I feel as the chronically ill must. This isn't living. It's surviving. Barely. Every minute is agony. I've got the vision-altering migraine and thirst-hunger of the dehydrated. The scale keeps dropping because my stomach can't hold on to anything, including water. My limbs feel so weak that it's surprising I haven't passed out while teaching or driving. Usually, I pride myself on gritting through sickness, refusing even ibuprofen, but now I call the doctor and beg for medicine.

"If you're still holding down some food," the nurses say, "then it's not severe enough to warrant IVs."

I can consider antinausea meds, but in a small percentage of pregnancies, there are risks to the fetus. I'm not willing to chance it. Day in and day out I think about fake-fainting so I'll be sent to the ER and get some kind of relief.

A horrible thought crosses my mind.

I don't want to be pregnant anymore. Not if it means feeling like this.

Chapter

23

I t is the year of the baby.

Seven, yes *SEVEN,* of my friends are pregnant. In Chicago, it's Tammy, Cailin, Gail, and Haley. In Massachusetts, it's Melissa and Jenn. In Guatemala, it's Michelle. Jenn and I joke that there must have been something in the waters of Lake Atitlan, seeing as how we and Michelle all got pregnant within six months of the writing retreat.

I know that I should wait to tell more people, but I spill my own good news to a few of my closest Chicago friends. Almost each one I tell has their own announcements or someone else's to share. And it seems as if August was a good sex month, because almost all of them are due within weeks of me.

On my drives to and from the university, I daydream about my Massachusetts friends and me meeting up for playdates— our kids crawling around together, us mothers bonding over the trials and tribulations of parenthood.

But, tonight, while reading my pregnancy handbook before bed, I come to the chapter on miscarriage. My eyes insist on traveling over the words—symptoms like cramping and bleeding, and the most troubling statistic: One out of every four women will suffer a miscarriage.

Seven friends plus me makes eight. That means that two of

us will lose our babies. I pray that because I am personally connected to these women, that they—that we—are safe, that this ratio doesn't apply to us.

But, of course, last October's events proved to me that everybody eventually becomes part of some tragic percentage, including me. And because Jamie and I have experienced firsthand what it's like to get too hopeful only to have that hope yanked away, I half-expect the very same thing to happen this time. I wonder, *Has IVF abducted the optimistic me that used to think everything would be OK? And by wishing, in my lowest moments, for this pain of pregnancy to end, am I provoking my uterus to miscarry?*

After setting the book down on my nightstand, I rub cocoa butter over my small-but-growing bump, and I look up at the ceiling.

I think of my friends and myself in terms of pictures on playing cards. I see all eight of our head shots spread out on a table. I pray to the omniscient power above, *Don't flip over my card. Please please please don't flip over my card. We've been through too much. I wouldn't be able to handle it. It would be the end of me.*

What would I do if I miscarried? I wonder. My brain shows flashes of me doing what I do best in stressful situations: fleeing—quitting my job, shutting everyone out. I'd move to somewhere like Guatemala, and hide away in a remote village on Lake Atitlan in a small hut of a home. I'd try to distract myself from the sorrow by learning a new language. Or maybe I'd move back to Chicago and let the city distract me. Would I be strong enough to take on Jamie's pain, too? I don't know. I fear that my deep despair would toxify every interaction with everyone around me. Such a loss, after all we've been through, would surely turn me crazy or inconsolable. I don't know which would be worse—to be permanently insane or permanently sad.

But I do know that if my card isn't flipped over, that means that someone else's will be.

Please don't flip any cards, I pray as I turn off my lamp.

Though, as of late, I usually fall asleep the second my head hits the pillow, tonight my eyes stay open long after I pull the covers over me. I can hear Jamie starting a movie downstairs in the living room. When he comes to bed two hours later, I'm still awake, eyebrows furrowed with fret. He kisses me and reaches over to rub my belly, but soon his snores boom through the room. I stare at the dark ceiling for another hour, worrying.

When I finally fall asleep, I dream. Vividly. In these sub-conscious visions, we have a baby girl whom I place in a dresser drawer. When I return to open the drawer, her body is deflated, like a plastic doll with all the air sucked out.

I go to the bathroom constantly, terrified that when I pull down my pants, I'll find blood spots in my underwear. My pre-vious fear of dying in my sleep for no reason has now been replaced with my fear of our baby dying at any time for no reason.

I don't want to worry anymore. I want to go back in time to when Jamie and I were newly married, when I felt oblivi-ously optimistic. Like every other naïve twenty-seven-year-old who hasn't truly been hardened by life, I thought that because my family had always struggled for money and my parents had always fought and I'd always been at odds with Mom, life had already dealt me my fair share of suffering. Anything that I'd achieved was through my own efforts, and, as my reward, I believed that the universe would just hand me everything for which I worked. I wasn't afraid to be happy, wasn't perpetually apprehensive that sorrow lurked around the corner.

What kind of pregnant person might I have been two years ago, before all of our heartbreak? Surely, I'd feel less guilty about my bliss and less worried about miscarriage.

IVF forever changed my outlook. It forever changed me. But maybe if it hadn't been IVF, it would have been some other incident. Maybe life needed to teach me a lesson about entitlement, about gratitude, and IVF was just the form it took.

The following weekend, on a vibrant October morning in my ninth week, Jamie and I go apple picking—one of my favorite fall activities—and I feel so wretched while we climb the hills that we have to call it quits after we've picked just a handful of Cortlands. I'm shivering and sweating and nauseous and hungry and throbbing and noodley. When we get home, I lie in bed and sob to Jamie, "I want to be hit by a bus. I just want this to end."

He rubs my arm quietly, but he looks at me the same way he did in the hospital last October when I feared dying in my sleep, like he's afraid I might soon need a straitjacket and a padded cell. I can see his brain spinning, and I know he's contemplating calling my doctor. I want to reassure him that I am not serious, but I can't. I hate that, once again, he has to take care of me. Sometimes, I feel so selfish that Jamie always has to be my rock.

I say this to Jamie now, and he shakes his head, shooing away the comment. "You're growing our baby," he says.

He sets me up on the couch and puts in the movie *Brides-maids* to cheer me up, but even this—one of my favorite movies—can't make me laugh. I sweat and shiver, layer blankets on top of me, then kick them off. We lie in the L of our sectional, my head in Jamie's lap. He presses his palm to my forehead to relieve the headache pressure. He gets me coconut water and orders a veggie pizza. I eat little bits, then moan and lie back down. Jamie presses my forehead again. He doesn't say much, just listens, rubs, presses, says, "I'm sorry you feel shitty, Nader."

Before I fell in love with Jamie, I used to think that love

was some grand gesture—some loud declaration, some big show. But love, at least in our relationship, is so much subtler than that. It's as small as a freckle. It's when I make over-easy eggs and blueberry tea for Jamie in the morning. It's how he automatically switches on the passenger seat heater for me when we take winter drives in his truck. It's how I sit in his lap after dinner and massage his scalp. It's how he stays with me now, just like he did after my emergency surgery, even though there are a million other things he could be doing.

After the movie, we stay on the couch and I skip ahead in *What to Expect When You're Expecting* to find out when this morning-sickness agony will end. It says that come the second trimester, the nausea should subside and my energy will return. *OK*, I think, *this is good news. Just five more weeks,* I think. *Just make it to Thanksgiving and you'll get relief.*

That night, after throwing up the pizza, I ponder why some of us get morning sickness and some of us don't. *Why is it that two of my pregnant Chicago friends feel totally fine?* I wonder.

I call up my Massachusetts friend, Tiffany. She's a mother of three kids under the age of five. If anyone can relate, she certainly can.

She says, "Just think of every day that you're sick as another day your baby is healthy."

That night, I find Jamie staring at our ultrasound photo on the fridge. He doesn't know I'm watching him from the doorway, and I see him place his finger to the little dinosaur that is our baby, gently stroking it. He shakes his head in wonder. He smiles so widely, I can feel the fullness of his heart from across the room.

And, I think, maybe that's how I'll survive this. Maybe it's not meds or IVs that I need, maybe it's an optimistic outlook and some awe. But what if my optimism turns into excitement, and my excitement climbs so high that if we were to miscarry, the fall from it would be devastating?

My bridesmaid dress is long and brown and one-shouldered and beautifully accentuates my teensy bump. As we pose for bridal-party pictures against the fall backdrop, I find myself unconsciously cupping my abdomen. In actuality, my belly merely looks bloated, but I'm cupping it anyway. Each time, I look around, hoping I haven't upset any of Kelly's bridesmaids.

When I walk down the aisle holding a bouquet of peach roses and orange daisies, I catch Jamie grinning at me from his place at the front of the tent with the other groomsmen. After the ceremony, when we link up and walk back down the aisle together, he kisses my temple, and says, "You look beautiful, wifey."

All the pregnancy clichés are true tonight—my unblemished skin glows and my hair lies in thick waves. I feel lovely. Still nauseous. Still headachy. But lovely.

In our couple's picture, Jamie leans down and kisses my stomach. My nose scrunches in delight. Still, I quickly force my face into neutral, afraid of being the same insensitive jerk that I was during the bachelorette party.

During dinner, Jamie dotes on me, making sure my water glass is always full. He wraps his arm around my shoulders and whispers in my ear. He knows most of the guests, so he introduces me to his high school acquaintances and family friends. He keeps his hand on my back and says, "This is my wife, Nadine," then touches my stomach, and adds, "and this is Baby Johnstone."

The more people he tells about our pregnancy, the more he makes me feel like I hold the power of the world in my belly. Still, I'm conscious of Kelly's friends. I don't want to them to overhear Jamie telling the story of the day I came to his office with the pregnancy test. But when I spot them in the crowd, they're busy dancing and posing with their spouses in the photo booth.

Shouldn't I be doing the same? I ask myself. *Aren't I allowed to be happy, too?* And a voice answers strongly back, *Yes.*

So, when I slow dance with Jamie, surrounded by twinkle lights and flickering candles, I lean into him. He places one hand in mine and the other on our baby. And I finally accept that it's OK for the world to see. Jamie twirls me, and my dress swirls around my ankles.

When he pulls me back, my belly touches him, connecting us.

Chapter

24

"You excited?" Jamie asks, passing me the baking soda. We're talking in the sunny kitchen, and I'm making Grandma Kenney's Irish bread to bring to Jamie's cousin's house for Thanksgiving.

"I thought this day would never come," I say. I still have to drink my peppermint tea to take the edge off my headaches and nausea, but, true to the pregnancy book's prediction, my first trimester has ended, and I've held down meals for a week. There's also the reassurance that because our baby made it through the risky first term, he or she is much more likely to develop smoothly from here on out.

Measuring cups and mixing bowls crowd our counters, summoning instant contentment. Into the batter I sprinkle cinnamon, nutmeg, and allspice. I pour in the vanilla, the milk, the raisins, then blend the ingredients with my bare hands the way Grandma Kenney used to.

"Do you have the printout?" I ask.

Jamie hands over a sheet of yellow paper, which I'll cut into strips that read: *This bread is ready to eat, but we've got another bun in the oven. Baby Johnstone due May 19.*

We walk down the stone path to Jamie's cousin's house,

and I carry a basket of individually wrapped bread slices. Each one is tied in a ribbon that bears the announcement strip. I'm wearing a purposely formfitting sweater dress and a belt above my bump, but I plan to keep my coat on until people read the message, then I'll do the big reveal.

Before we open the door, Jamie kisses me, and says, "I love how proud you are."

I think back to last Thanksgiving, me crying over my sister-in-law's pregnancy, how I thought this day would never come for us.

Now it's here. And Jamie's right. I am proud. I am actually just proud. Not sick and proud. Not worried and proud. I am simply, wonderfully, proud.

With that, we step into his cousin's house. We inhale the smell of sweet potatoes and pumpkin pie.

And we pass out our bread.

The next couple of weeks are as bright and glittery as the Christmas lights lining our windows. My nausea disappears, and despite my new Oreo fixation, I even crave healthy foods. My headaches still hang around, but they're much less brutal than before.

Most exciting, though, is that Kelly is pregnant. It seems she and Mikey are in the rare percentage of people who have absolutely no trouble conceiving on demand. I'm giddy with the desire for us to share all of our milestones together. I meet up with Kelly and her maid of honor, Melissa, at the Providence Place Mall. As we eat lunch and compare our small, medium, and large bellies, we realize that we are each in a different trimester. Kelly is in her first. I'm in my second, and Melissa is in her third. I feel so lucky to be able to share this experience with them.

"Are you burping all the time?" I ask. Melissa nods and says, "Don't worry, that'll be the least of your concerns. Just wait till you get kicked in the ribs."

"I have so much to look forward to," Kelly says, and we laugh for the next two hours over the strange gifts that come with carrying a baby.

During my lunch break the following week, while sitting in the teacher's lounge eating minestrone soup, I feel fizzing inside my abdomen on my left side. It feels like carbonated bubbles floating to the top of a shaken soda bottle. I think it might be gas, but then I feel a swipe in the same spot, and I realize that it's our baby.

The realness of it moving inside of me is indescribable. It's like my baby and I share some kind of secret language. It can communicate to me without anybody else knowing.

How do you react when you're engulfed in pure happiness?

I pause for a moment with my hands on my middle and look around, taking in the moment. The faculty lounge is in a loft area in the library. On the lower levels, students type papers and read textbooks. Librarians help students use the research computers. I think back to my time spent in the hospital last year—how my life seemed to stop while the world kept going. I was angry at the universe. But now, a little over a year later, the same thing is happening. I am paused while the rest of the world keeps rotating, but this time, the moment is the high-light of a lifetime.

My heart feels the same love I did the night I met Jamie and the day we got married, the same appreciation as when I sat on the dock in Guatemala wrapped in my blue shawl.

I press ever so lightly on the same spot as the swipe. In return, my stomach fizzes, as if the baby is saying, *I'm here, Mama. I'm strong, Mama. I love you, Mama.*

I celebrate by planning the nursery decor via Pinterest—gray nurseries, yellow accents, woodland themes, tepee reading tents.

Jamie laughs and says, "Who's the tepee really for, you or the baby?"

I am feeling so good about everything that I compose an email to my pregnant friends in Illinois to check up on them. But just as I'm about to press send, a friend calls sounding tense. She tells me that both Tammy's and Gail's babies stopped developing. They were the two out of my eight pregnant friends that did not have morning sickness and the two to have their cards flipped. They also both lost their babies at the beginning of their second trimesters, a time period that I always thought marked a transition into safety and guaranteed survival. I feel horrible for them and guilty for still being pregnant when they aren't.

Another terrifying thought: *What if the stats are off, and the rest of us are still in danger, too?*

As I hold the phone, speechless, my own sweet baby kicks. But now I feel like I can't decode our language anymore. Is it really saying *I'm strong* or is it actually saying *Something's wrong?*

Chapter

25

My folders and books all go into a pile as I transform the second bedroom into the baby's room. I can't believe that now, two and a half years after we bought our home, we finally get to turn this nook into the nursery I imagined. Soon we'll get to place little toys on the bookshelves and a glider under the skylight.

It's a lovely room—sunlit with a view of the backyard trees. It's small without feeling cramped. When we first moved here, right before we got married, I turned it into my writing room. It would be temporary, until I got pregnant. With its slanted ceilings and built-in desk, the room looked exactly like the space Louisa May Alcott had used for penning her novels. And though I filled the drawers with notebooks and pinned inspirational quotes on my bulletin board, I've only written here a couple of times since we moved in. It's too quiet, and I end up going to cafés instead, though the nearest Starbucks is a twenty-minute drive. I'm nostalgic for my grad school days when there was an Argo Tea right down the block from my studio apartment.

Since my books and daybed take up all the space, we haven't been able to do much in this room besides paint. The whole process of stowing my things and replacing them with our child's possessions feels symbolic, a transition into a life where someone else's needs will be more important than my own. I just hope that putting my novel pages away in Rubbermaids isn't a premonition for the future. I worry that once the baby gets here, I'll lose myself, and my writing career will disintegrate. Who am I if I am not a writer, if I am not always striving toward something? Part of my personality is that I am always in progress. It's something that I get from Mom. Though she never went to college, she started off as a bank teller and was promoted to manager. Then, in my teens, she changed careers to become a personal trainer and, later, a masseuse. She is always pursuing her next certification. A couple years ago, when I decided to go to El Salvador alone to teach an English course, some people balked at the idea, asking why I'd want to go by myself. But Mom understood. Having grown up on the South Side of Chicago with three brothers, she had learned to fend for herself, and she instilled that same self-sufficiency in Dana and me.

I use that same determined energy now to clear the room. Little by little, I fill bins with my old journals and literary magazines and heave them onto the top shelf of my closet. I know I should be careful about lifting heavy things, but I feel good. I feel strong. Plus, I find it a bit ridiculous when pregnant women make their husbands carry their purses. Each time, I think, *Really? Come on.* Now that I'm not nauseous anymore, I want to be as low maintenance of a pregnant wife as possible.

By the time Jamie comes home from work, the entire room is emptied, and all he has to do is move the daybed into the basement. I look at the gray walls and empty shelves, and I think about how, soon, Jamie will put down the new carpet and assemble the crib.

We will bring our baby home to this room.

I show Jamie the empty shelves and drawers, expecting him to be impressed, but he looks worried. "You should have waited for me to help you," he says. "Where did you put all the stuff?" he asks. I point to the top shelves of the closet where I lined up the Rubbermaids.

"How did you get them up there?" he asks.

"I lifted them," I say.

Jamie looks at me, then at my belly. "You should have waited for me to help you," he repeats.

My cheeks grow red. "They weren't that heavy," I say.

My defensive brain grumbles that Jamie is treating me like an invalid. *I may be growing a child,* I reason, *but I'm still capable of doing things.* I walk downstairs to the bathroom, turning on the fan to cover my angry whispers.

And then I pull down my underwear.

There are light brown spots on the cotton.

Dried blood spots.

My hand shakes as I wipe myself. There is the slightest twinge of brown on the toilet paper.

This can't be happening, I think.

When I emerge from the bathroom, I can't even look Jamie in the eye, I feel so ashamed. He's in the middle of making ground turkey for tacos. As I explain that it's nothing, just some little spots, he becomes very still, very quiet. We both know what hangs in the air.

If I caused a miscarriage . . .

With trembling fingers, I dial the on-call doctor. Jamie stands beside me in the dining room, listening on speakerphone.

"If it's not accompanied by cramping and fresh bleeding, then you don't need to come to the ER tonight," she says. "But just to be sure, come to the hospital tomorrow morning for an ultrasound."

I should be relieved, but I'm terrified. Guilt pours over me by the bucketload.

There's one thing I know for sure: If I miscarry, I will never forgive myself. Jamie wouldn't forgive me either, and he would have every right not to.

During dinner, I hold my breath to concentrate on the baby's movements. But even when I do feel the fizz and the swipe of its limbs, I worry that these are the kicks of a dying fetus.

Why do I always push myself so hard? I've already seen what it cost me last October. Why, oh why haven't I learned?

After barely touching my meal, I get ready for bed. Jamie heads into the living room, where he stares at the TV, though I know his brain is elsewhere. I can't bear to meet his eyes. I know his pupils would be wide with questions. *"What's wrong with you? Why couldn't you just take it easy? Why couldn't you ask for help? What are you trying to prove?"*

It's the same look I've given Mom on countless occasions. During my childhood, when Dana and I would play, Mom would always be hopping from laundry to dishes, and I just wanted her to relax for once. The few times Mom cried, she quickly blotted her tears, and I thought, "Who are you trying to be strong for?" I wanted her to be open and vulnerable. On the occasions I tried to explain something to Mom, like how to use the computer, she'd quickly snap that she could do it herself. I wanted to tell her that it was OK to ask for help.

And here I am, her exact replica.

How can it be that the same tenacity that propels us forward is the very thing that costs us so much?

It seems to take hours for the technician to ready the machine and lube up my stomach. Usually they warm the gel, but because we're the first patients, the glob is cold and alarming when it touches my skin. Jamie looks distressed. Instead of exuding hives and sweat as I do, he sits, unmoving and mute.

The room itself feels like a womb—confined and dark. It's almost cozy, but I'm afraid, in a matter of minutes, we're going to find out terrible news that will make it feel like a coffin.

The young technician grabs the wand and lowers it to my belly. She's quiet, and I wonder if she already has a sense that we're doomed. I close my eyes for a second, afraid of seeing our lifeless child on the screen.

I feel the tech press the wand near my belly button and hear her tap at the keys on the machine.

One sentence plays over and over again in my mind.

It's my fault. It's all my fault.

The technician wiggles the wand.

Is she trying to jostle our motionless baby?

I can't open my eyes.

If the baby isn't moving, if I have caused its death, I will go mad with guilt. I will not be able to live with myself. How could my life possibly go on if I have killed our precious child because I was too stubborn to ask for help?

Please let it move, I beg. *Please let it be alive.*

Then I feel something.

Jamie squeezes my hand, and I open my eyes.

On the screen I see what I'm feeling. The glorious kick of our baby.

It's having a dance party inside my stomach, as if to reassure me that not only is it doing OK, it's a bundle of energy.

Tears burn my eyes, and the creases of Jamie's are moist, too.

We both exhale a long, slow breath.

"We've got quite a mover," the technician says, and we laugh.

"Just like its mama," Jamie chirps. How quickly he has forgiven me. How quickly the moment has tipped toward the best possible outcome. What would be happening right now if the baby hadn't kicked, hadn't moved?

I stare at the screen, shocked at how much our baby has grown in just a matter of weeks. It takes up much more of my uterus now and has long limbs and a potbelly. I want to see Raya-Geo's face, but even when the tech switches to 3-D, the baby's nose and mouth are buried in my body.

Although we've crossed one hurdle, my cervix is the next cause for concern. Is it thinning? Is that part of why I bled? And if so, will I need permanent bed rest for the next five months?

The technician zooms in on the small gray spot of my cervix. She measures it with the cursor and smiles.

"Looks good," she says, then adds, "Do you want to know the sex?"

Jamie and I nod, synchronized.

"Can you tell us?" I ask.

She moves the wand down toward my pubic bone, to the right a little, and zooms in. The cursor travels over our baby's bum and magnifies the area.

Then the tech points to a nub of flesh between its skinny legs.

"It's a boy," she says.

Our mouths drop open. Before the technician leaves the room, she prints out pictures of our son.

Our son. Our Geo.

How is it that the visions I had years ago of our boy were actually correct? I think back to the framed picture of Jamie as a toddler, of the blue thread we chose in Italy for the Vitello bib, of how, during IVF, when I envisioned one embryo surviving, it was Geo.

All along, did my subconscious know what lay in our future?

Jamie leans down and kisses me repeatedly. He looks like he might run down the hall and shout the news to everyone. "There's a miniature you in there," I tell him as I point to my belly.

"I can't believe it," he says again and again.

"Look at those flippers," I say, propping myself up on my elbows as Jamie holds the pictures in front of us. "Those are definitely your feet," I say, laughing.

The doctor is overbooked, and we have to wait a while, so the technician comes back in the room and does another ultrasound so we can have extra glimpses of our baby boy.

I wish medical personnel knew how much their attitude and gestures affect their patients. This technician didn't have to come back in and visit us. She could have used the time to check email or browse Facebook. Instead, she gave two giddy parents an amazing gift. I wonder if my theory of balance is valid, and this appointment is making up for some of the awful ones we've had over the past two years.

Finally the doctor—a short, wiry guy with glasses—comes in and puts the wand to my stomach once more.

"Yep, that's a dingus," he says, zeroing in on the penis.

Surprised at the slang, Jamie and I laugh hard and my belly shakes, making the image on the screen bounce.

The doctor smiles, and I like that he doesn't take himself too seriously.

"Alright," he says, handing me a towel so I can wipe off the goop. "So, just to be on the safe side, no strenuous activity and no sex for you two. I'll see you back here in two weeks to check your cervix again."

When he turns on the lights and shuts the door, Jamie helps me off the padded table.

"You know we're going to have to call him Dr. Dingus from now on," I joke.

"Exactly what I was thinking," Jamie says.

We laugh some more and hug each other hard.

"I love you George James Johnstone the fourth," I say to Jamie. "And the fifth," I say to my stomach.

And to the universe, I promise, *I will learn. I will learn to take it easy. I will learn to ask for help.*

Chapter

26

It is the end of the semester, and I only have one workshop left to teach on Saturday. With piles of term papers stacked before me, all I can do is close the classroom door and kick off my flats. I am so ready for a break, and so are my dress pants, which strain at my bulging waist. Unbuttoning them feels as good as changing into sweatpants at the end of a long day.

The classroom windows reveal the gray December sky, but I just feel lucky that this winter has been a mild one, with no snow yet. The bigger highlight of this day, though, is that we are picking Mom and Dana up from the airport tonight.

I wonder if they will seem like strangers. When I left Illinois, I was on the cusp of twenty-five and newly in love. Dana was a sophomore in college, partying and free of responsibility. Mom and I were constantly fighting with each other to be understood.

Now Dana's an adult with a real job, living in a city apartment with her boyfriend. And on the phone, Mom seems different, too—more submissive toward me, regarding me as a grown woman. I wonder how it will be for Mom to stay at our house for the first time and see me as a future mother. She hasn't witnessed the person I've become over the past four and a half years. How will I seem to her?

Though I feel grateful for what the years away have done

for me—made me more confident, more independent—I also wonder what roles I've neglected. Dana hasn't had a big sister in a long time, and Mom must feel like she has one daughter instead of two.

I haven't celebrated Christmas with Mom and Dana since I moved away, and, though we're a week early, I'm desperate to do so. I didn't appreciate it as a kid, but now I yearn for all the traditions from Mom's annual Christmas Eve party—fried chicken and mostaccioli, Uncle Frank dressing up as Santa. I loved how Dana and I got to open one gift early, which was always a pair of new pajamas that we'd wear to bed that night. We didn't sing carols by the fire like the March girls did in the *Little Women* Christmases I pined for, but I realize, now, that Mom put great effort into getting our rowdy Chicago family together and making the holiday memorable for us.

As soon as Mom and Dana arrive at the airport, they sprint out to our car—Dana relaxed in yoga pants, Mom fashionable in jeans and boots. But Mom looks different. Her hair is shorter. She has reading glasses on her head. There's something about her that seems less intimidating. When I step out of Jamie's truck to hug them, both sets of eyes light up, and they reach immediately for my bump.

I want the baby's gender to be a surprise for them when they go to the ultrasound with us tomorrow. So, I'm trying hard to recite everything in my head before I speak. Everything I want to say involves "he." *Wait till you see him tomorrow. He's so cute.* It's very strange to say "it" now that we know our baby is a boy.

Jamie and Mom hug, and any old tension that may have existed between them about my move to Massachusetts is nonexistent in the moment.

"Congratulations, Dad," Mom says. Jamie grins and lifts her suitcase into the trunk.

Mom cups my stomach in her hands. "You're still tiny," she says.

"Well, that's good," I say, "because I don't feel tiny."

Our breaths come out in icy puffs, and cars line up behind ours to pick up friends and family members. Good airport etiquette would call for hurling the rest of the luggage into the trunk and driving away, but we stand there, suspended in time. It's the first time my own mother has seen me with child. It's strange and lovely all at once. Though I'm almost thirty, sometimes I still feel like an imposter, like I'll be discovered unfit to raise a child, and of all people's opinions, Mom's is the one that matters the most to me. *Does she believe in me?* I wonder. *Does she think I'll be a good mother?*

The way that she looks at me, I can't tell if she's just in awe that she's going to be a grandma or if she's proud that I'm going to be a mom.

When Dana presses her hands to my bump, I instinctively say, "He's quite the kicker."

They both squeal, "He!?" and I say, "Shit!"

Jamie shakes his head and laughs at me.

"Smooth, Nader," he says. "Real smooth."

During the fifty-minute ride home, we make plans for all of the Christmasy things we'll do this weekend—pick out a tree, make pies, decorate gingerbread houses, maybe even take a picture with Santa at the mall. I'm giddy with a feeling that I can't name—one that's the opposite of homesickness.

I also cannot wait to do baby-related stuff with them. I want to buy bibs for Geo that say things like "My auntie is the best" and "Grandma's little guy." I also need to do some very necessary maternity clothes shopping. Because my old, irrational IVF fears have convinced me that if I buy too many belly-paneled outfits, I'll jinx everything, I've been wearing baggy clothes and hand-me-downs. But now it's time. Not only are my pants straining at the seams, I've made it to eighteen weeks and have a confirmed baby boy growing inside of me. I can finally relax a bit and accept that this is really happening. Jamie and I are really going to have a baby.

When we pull into our driveway, I hold my breath and await Mom's reaction. I want her to be proud of the home that Jamie and I have created. I wonder if she will notice that the house's layout resembles that of our old house on the South Side.

When I was fourteen and Dana was nine, we left that South Side A-frame for a suburban split-level, but I still think of our Chicago two-story as my childhood home. When Jamie and I were looking at houses, I kept saying that I wanted stairs that led to the bedrooms, like the home of my youth. But unlike Mom and Dad, who left up the previous owner's wallpaper and paneling, Jamie and I have remodeled almost every room of our house to make it our own.

Tessa greets us at the slider, tail swinging. She shimmies between Dana's short legs, lifting her right off the ground.

As I open the door, I feel as if I am giving Mom a tour not of our house, but of the person I've become over the last few years. We enter through the sunporch, and I explain that this is where I read and take naps on Sunday afternoons. This is where Jamie and I eat when the weather's nice. In our yellow kitchen, I point to the brightly colored art that my students gave me in El Salvador.

In the dining room, I show Mom and Dana the wood floors and light fixture that Jamie installed himself. In the living room, they see the old cast-iron stove and the wooden beams that hang the lanterns we've collected during our weekend trips around New England.

"It's cozy, isn't it?" Dana says.

Mom stands in the middle of the room, looking at all of the 1907 detail.

"It's so welcoming," she says as she touches my arm. The spot tingles even after her fingers leave it. And though this room is the opposite of our South Side living room, there is plenty of evidence of my Chicago childhood. Unlike when I first moved to Massachusetts and couldn't bear to be reminded of the Midwest, now dressers and walls display photos of my entire life, not just my life in Massachusetts. The staircase shelves showcase pictures from my youth. Mom spots them and fishes her reading glasses out of her hair to get a better look. There's the photo of her with Dana and me on Halloween. Mom is dressed as a Hershey's bar, Dana is a flower, and I am a tube of toothpaste. Mom made all of our costumes. Though she wasn't much of a sewer, she could work magic with duct tape and a glue gun. The next picture shows Mom reading to me and Dana in my bed. My New Kids on the Block poster of Jordan Knight covers the wall behind my headboard.

Now, Dana, Mom, and I crowd around the picture, laughing at Mom's eighties perm and my NKOTB obsession.

"You look so young there," Dana says to Mom.

"That's because I was," Mom says.

I do the quick calculations and am shocked at the results: In that picture, I am seven, Dana is two, and Mom is a mere twenty-six years old. No wonder Mom was always escaping to the bathroom for cigarettes and rare moments of peace.

After we look at the rest of the pictures, Jamie puts the suitcases away and lights the stove. I make hot chocolate and play Christmas music. We all sit around the living room as the lantern lights twinkle and the gas stove warms us. I take sips from my mug and absorb the joy of being able to have my family in my living room with me.

We stay up way past my 8:00 p.m. bedtime, talking about the nursery and my baby shower coming up in April. Mom is excited to take a tour of the maternity floor after my ultra-sound tomorrow.

Dana lies on the sectional couch under a blanket, rubbing her feet together, as she used to when she was young. It's comforting to see that even though she has grown into an adult, there are still parts of her that are familiar.

Mom perches on the edge of the couch and slides her reading glasses on to decipher the candy-cane nametags taped to gifts she brought. I'm still not used to this. The glasses make her seem older, gentler. It's hard to pinpoint, but there's something consoling in the fact that the same woman who never wanted help finally requires just the slightest bit of assistance. It makes Mom seem more vulnerable somehow. And there's something else. Her manicured nails catch my eye as she sorts through the gifts. Mom rarely treated herself to anything when we were young besides trips to the Kohl's clearance rack. I'm happy that she finally has the means to indulge a bit now that she's not worried about supporting Dana and me.

She hands out presents—a coral-colored scarf for me, a button-down shirt for Jamie. She even has a monkey ornament for Geo. And, true to tradition, she gives Dana and me each a pair of pajamas.

In some ways, Mom is still the same. She slips out to the backyard for a cigarette. She drains her coffee and talks a million miles per hour. But her excitement over Geo is palpable. I realize that, like every other pregnant woman on the planet, I am starting to appreciate Mom more now that I am expecting my own child. It's hard for me to believe that Mom went through this sort of alien abduction that people call pregnancy when she was just nineteen, stranded in Hawaii in a volatile marriage. At my age now—twenty-nine—Mom already had a ten-year-old. She sacrificed so that I'd have an extra decade to play and travel and get an education and be independent.

Fond memories of her hosting birthday parties and bringing us to bowling excursions come back to me now as I acknowledge how much sacrifice went into raising us. I feel a deep desire to write her a book-length apology letter for any strife I've ever caused her.

I just hope that she can sense my appreciation from my extra smiles.

Maybe she's feeling more bonded, too, because, on our way up to bed, she hugs me and says, "I can't wait to meet my grandson tomorrow!"

I hug her back and we hold each other tight, our first quality hug in a long, long time. I feel seven again, like I'm sitting in the bathroom as she wraps my hair around a curling iron, taking great care with each strand. When I think of Mom nurturing me, this is the memory I always come back to: us in the Pepto-pink bathroom of our old house on the South Side. Usually, the bathroom was Mom's sanctuary. It's where she went to smoke her Benson and Hedges Gold 100s. She had an ashtray on the counter that Grandpa had brought back from Vegas and featured a pair of dice. And Mom would sit on the toilet, smoking. That way, if anyone barged in on her, she could claim that she was still using the bathroom. She'd stay in there for twenty minutes at a time, just staring at the pink walls, smoking. But on Saturdays, if we were going somewhere, she allowed me into her fortress. I sat on the closed toilet, staring at her sweatshirt as she curled my hair. Mom spent hours preparing me for outings and parties, as if the completeness of her love depended on the bounce of my curls, the straightness of my part. She lit cigarettes that she forgot to smoke, and I felt satisfied when she held my comb in between her teeth instead of her Benson and Hedges. I smiled when the ash burned down to the filter, covering the dice on the ashtray, because it meant that I was Mom's highest priority in that moment.

Because she rarely splurged on herself, Mom always wore the same sweatshirt that read, "Guess knitwear goes mad for plaid," and the same heart necklace. I stared at the tiny gold heart pendant, watching it move as she coiled my hair around the curling iron.

Later, my uncle told me that, as a teenager, Mom had stolen the necklace from her friend. I couldn't imagine it.

"Oh, your Mom was quite the rebel back in the day," he said. Mom was so straitlaced during my youth—rarely drinking, rarely going out—that it seemed we were talking about someone else. Then again, Mom had gotten married shortly after her high school graduation and followed her new husband across the US for his military career. She missed a month of birth control, and suddenly, I was a tiny worry in her womb.

I imagine that her call home to announce the news wasn't nearly as joyous as mine was. But instead of yelling, Grandma uttered her famous saying, "When there's a will, there's a way."

In my teen years, I asked Mom what had stopped her from having an abortion. She said that, one afternoon, she had the phone book in her lap and started to dial the clinic, but she couldn't complete the call, and that was that.

"I was an accident," I sometimes joked. But Mom reassured me that I was the best kind of accident. "I love you more than life itself," she would say in our rare moments of sentimentality. She would hug me, and I could feel her heart pendant pressing into my chest.

Tonight, I fall asleep with an image in my head—me in five months, sitting up in a sunlit hospital bed, holding out my arms toward my just-delivered son, who is swaddled in a blue blanket. My skin is dewy, and my wavy hair spreads over my bare shoulders like a shawl. Mom strokes my hair as I embrace my son.

The next morning, as Jamie drives us to the ultrasound appointment, Mom, Dana, and I pull out our makeup bags in unison. Synchronized, we open our compacts and study ourselves in the little mirrors. Dana is the first to notice. "Weird," she says, laughing. All three of us are holding our compacts in our left hand and applying lip gloss with our right.

When Mom twists the cap off of her Cover Girl foundation, the Noxzema smell morphs time. Dana and I are kids again, cruising down Pulaski in our Buick Regal as Mom swipes the ivory foundation across her cheeks. Her right knee guides the steering wheel.

Something about this strikes me, now—how, over the last four and a half years, every time Jamie drove, and I applied my makeup in the passenger seat, I did it in the exact fashion as Mom had to her own face. And eight hundred miles away in the Midwest, Dana and Mom were also doing the same ritualistic cosmetic application as I was in Massachusetts. How far I've moved away from them and how close I've still stayed.

In the cramped ultrasound room, the four of us stare at the gray screen and the technician squirts goop onto the wand. Dana has never been to an ultrasound before, and she stares curiously, trying to make out what the tech is doing with the tangle of machinery before her.

Mom rubs my foot, and Dana says, "I'm gonna see my nephew!"

Cherish this, I think. *This is what I've been missing.* It's amazing how this little boy inside of me, whom none of us has ever met, can already bring about so much love and attention.

The gel is warm and sticky on my stomach, but the wand feels a bit hard as it rolls across my abdomen from my rib cage to my pubic bone.

Does it hurt Geo? I wonder. *Could the sound waves make him deaf? Does he even have ears yet?*

Before we can try to get a good look at the baby, the technician must first examine his limbs and organs. In the movies, when a pregnant character gets an ultrasound, it's all about the emotions—*"Look, there's your baby,"* the tech says, then the parents cry happily. But in real life, it's all about the measurements. Is his cranium radius normal? What about the length of the spine? The tech spends most of her time dragging the pointer vertically and horizontally across each of Geo's body parts and then pressing enter to record height and width. You never know from the technicians' neutral expressions if something's wrong.

"The doctor will discuss everything with you," they say each time.

Still, I always try to read their faces as they record numbers. *Was that a frown? What did that squint mean? Is my baby normal? Please tell me he's normal.*

We're quiet as the tech surveys Geo's limbs, and it's much less exciting than I anticipated. So, we play the who-can-identify-the-correct-organ game. "Is that the stomach?" Jamie asks, and I say, "I think that's the bladder."

The whole time, Geo messes with us by kicking and flipping so that the technician has to swirl the wand around for the right angle. But then the cursor moves to the heart, and I hold my breath, hoping that Geo will stay in place so we can hear the cadence of his pulse. The tech clicks a button and the screen switches to a graph of the beats per minute. Then she clicks the audio. That's when we finally get the emotional experience we had hoped for. The rhythmic gallop plays over the speakers. It's loud and steady and strong and magnificent.

Mom's breath catches in her throat. Dana whispers, "Oh my god," and dabs at her eyes with her sleeve.

"Isn't it awesome?" I say. "Hearing it makes it so real."

When the audio clip is over, I want the technician to play it again, but, having concluded the ultrasound, she stands up and prints off pictures.

218 Nadine Kenney Johnstone

We thank her, but she remains stone-faced and says that the doctor will be in soon.

I prop myself onto my elbows, and everyone crowds around me as we look at the pictures.

"Unbelievable," Mom says, shaking her head in amazement.

In the glossy black-and-whites, Geo looks like an old man, complete with potbelly and skinny legs.

When the doctor—Dr. Dingus—finally comes in, I expect the same jokey demeanor as last time, but he's all business.

He applies more gel and persistently rolls the wand around one side of my belly, as if he's looking for something. He squints at the screen and points the cursor at Geo's bladder.

He zooms in.

I wait for him to tell us how he's never seen anything like our son—that Geo is stronger and smarter than any other baby he's ever seen. I want him to tell me that I'll probably deliver early because Geo is just so developmentally advanced.

Instead, he turns away from the screen, looks at Jamie and me over his glasses, and takes a breath.

"I have a few things to talk to you about," he says. "And I need to know if you'd like me to speak to you two privately."

Confused, I stare at him, and he glances at Mom and Dana, implying that, if I'd like, he can ask them to leave the room.

This isn't good, I think. *He has bad news. This can't be happening.* My face goes pale. Fainting feels inevitable. Jamie's face flushes to a deep shade of purple; his pulse pounds in his eyes.

"They can stay," I say as calmly as possible, when I really want to say, *Just spit it the fuck out. What the hell is wrong with our baby?*

Mom gently squeezes my toe to show that she's here supporting me. Dana rubs my ankle. But I can see in their faces, and in Jamie's, that everyone is terrified.

With his cursor, the doctor points and commentates:

"Enlarged bladder."

"Distended kidneys."

"Two-vessel umbilical cord."

"Swollen genitals."

He says that though my initial integrative screening came back negative for Down syndrome and other genetic disorders, these are characteristics of trisomy 13, and we need to talk to a genetic counselor so I can get tested.

"It's a small chance, but . . ." His voice trails off.

He also says that he believes there is a blockage that's hindering Geo's ability to urinate. We need to go to Children's Hospital as soon as possible.

"If the baby can't urinate," he says, "it's detrimental."

He repositions his glasses nervously.

Air escapes me. A ball of dough clogs my windpipe. Hot tears stream down to my ears. Silent sobs heave my body. I feel like I'm in a casket at my own funeral with everyone looking down at me and crying.

"I need to sit up," I growl. "I need to sit up. Now."

Jamie pulls me up, and the table paper crunches underneath me. The goop gets all over my pants as my stomach presses against my thighs.

"Why?" I ask the doctor, as if it's something he can actually control. "Why can't I just have a normal pregnancy? We've already been through so much."

Jamie shifts from foot to foot and shoves his hands into his pockets. His chest is so puffed with anger that he looks like he could heave the ultrasound machine across the room.

We're escorted down the hallway to meet the genetic counselor, and I ask Mom and Dana to wait in the lobby. If we're told that our baby is doomed, I can't bear to see the sadness in their eyes. As we step into the office, Jamie and I instinctively reach for each other's hand.

The genetic counselor—a sneezing woman wearing an orthopedic leg boot—invites us to sit at a small cluttered table. Her bad immune system and bad fortune feel contagious. I Purell my hand after shaking hers.

As she repeatedly blows her nose, we fill out consent forms to have genetic tests for trisomy 13, 18, and 21.

The counselor gives vague descriptions of trisomy 13: "Worse than Down syndrome" and "Most babies don't survive."

We ask a series of questions to which she gives the same answer: "We won't know until we get the blood work."

"Most trisomy 13 babies have strawberry-shaped brains," she says, "and your baby does not. I can't say for sure," she adds, "but it seems unlikely that he has it."

She smiles ever so slightly, as if this tiny nugget of reassurance will make all our fears disappear. But then she ends the appointment with these parting words:

"If you test positive," she says, wiping her nose with a Kleenex, "you'll have until twenty-four weeks gestation to decide your course of action."

I frown, confused, until I realize that "course of action" means "to abort or not."

With that, she hobbles to the door to show us out of her office.

"You can get your blood drawn today," she says, "and we'll call you in two weeks with the news."

Two weeks? I think. *With all of today's technology, you mean to tell me that labs can't produce faster results? We really have to wait two whole weeks to find out whether our child is ill-fated? We have to sit and wonder for two weeks whether we will have to abort our own child?*

After the blood draw, we join Mom and Dana and file into the hallway to wait for the elevator. Should we still go up to the maternity floor for a tour?

But why? I ask myself. *Why would we want to see the delivery rooms when I might never deliver our son?*

I press the down arrow to the parking garage.

Jamie and I wait, gripping each other's hands tightly. It feels like if we let go, we'll both dissolve into the atmosphere. I shake my head and ask why this is happening to us. "What lesson is this supposed to teach us?" I ask Mom and Dana. "How can we abort our own baby when we've already heard his heartbeat?"

Because they can't answer, they just hug me. Mom holds me like I am her little girl. Dana squeezes me as if she is my big sister.

On the long ride home, Jamie's anxiety manifests into manic talking. He becomes a Massachusetts tour guide, rambling about landmarks to Mom and Dana the entire ride while I sit quietly, staring out the window at the houses we pass.

There are children in those houses, I think. *We will never have children in our own house.*

I close my eyes and wish to disappear.

Instinctively, my palm rests on my stomach. Then, realizing it, I pull my hand away. The long weekend stretches ahead, full of activities centered around a baby that might not ever be born. I decide that, tomorrow, we are not going anywhere near a Babies "R" Us or a maternity clothes section. I can already feel my brain severing the pathways that make any associations with "baby" and "pregnant."

I feel the same deep sadness I did when we lost our two transferred embryos, except this time, it's a million times worse. We're not losing a ball of cells. We're losing a fully formed four-month-old fetus with a brain and a beating heart. I know that, from now on, if anyone mentions Geo, I will have to redirect the conversation. I have to believe I am not pregnant.

As we park outside a restaurant for dinner, Children's

Hospital calls me. We remain in the truck, and I put the phone on speaker.

"The urine reflux and the distended kidneys—it's called hydronephrosis," the nurse says.

She explains that there are different levels of severity, and that, every once in a great while, these things correct themselves. I ask how severe Geo's hydronephrosis is, but she can't say for sure until they ultrasound me. When I schedule the appointment, we're urged to get in as soon as possible next week, even if that means missing work. The urgency of the appointment further heightens the seriousness of the situation.

The nurse recommends doing some research on hydronephrosis in the meantime.

I know that there is no way I'm looking up Geo's condition or else the words and images will occupy my every thought.

In my visor mirror, I see Mom Googling it on her phone and frowning.

"Have a good weekend," the nurse says before we hang up.

Right, I think.

"Don't look it up," Mom says as she shoves her phone into her purse.

"I wasn't planning on it," I say, then open the door and step out into the cold.

If I did search hydronephrosis, I'd see words like: renal and sexual dysfunction, permanent kidney damage, end-stage renal disease, and poor long-term prognosis.

And if that didn't freak me out enough, and I Googled trisomy 13, I'd see: heart defects, brain and spinal cord abnormalities, underdeveloped eyes, extra fingers or toes, cleft lip, cleft palate, and weak muscle tone.

Worst of all, I'd see this: if they survive in utero, infants with trisomy 13 usually die within the first months of life.

Chapter

27

have an obsession with scarves. They serve two functional purposes—to hide my nervous hives and to spruce up the handful of trendy outfits that I rotate through every week. But there's more to it than that. Scarves are my adult security blanket. I started wearing them when I moved out east, when I was trying to embark on the unknown. I wore silk scarves to job interviews, cotton scarves to dinner parties where I knew no one besides Jamie. Something about the weight of the fabric on my chest reassured me.

When we first moved into our house, Jamie hung two rows of hooks in the guest bedroom for my scarves. Upon entering the room, there is the rainbow of them lined up, looking like a wall of happiness.

The morning after our ultrasound, I have to teach one last Saturday ESL class, so I need that happiness and reassurance more than anything. As much as my students always cheer me up, I just want to curl up in a corner.

Mom and Dana stir when I knock on the guest bedroom door, and as Tess licks their faces, I climb into bed between them.

"I don't want to go to work," I say. My brain comes up with a list of excuses I can use to cancel class.

Mom rubs my arm.

"I don't want to go," I repeat.

"I know," Mom says. She lists the positives: "It's only a couple of hours. You love your students. This is your passion. It's the last class of the semester." I nod and stand, afraid of getting choked up if Mom looks me in the eye.

From my rows of scarves, I choose the coral-colored one that Mom gave me as a Christmas gift the other night, hoping that the orange hues will brighten this depressing day.

After hugging Mom and Dana goodbye, I drive the forty minutes to the university with the radio off. Dread fills the car like thick tar, swallowing me. There are only a handful of students in the class—all women—and each week they ask me about my pregnancy. Their excitement usually thrills me, giving me an excuse to brag to a captive audience. But today, I fear their questions.

Students wearing puffy coats carry trays of food into the ESL building, but I remain in my car, heat and worries on full blast. *What will happen when they ask me about Geo? Will I dissolve into despair before their very eyes? Will I even be able to teach?*

The first thing I see when I walk into the room are presents lined up on the front desk. The table by the window displays plates of food, including pan de queso, my favorite Brazilian snack. The women cheer when I walk in the door. Some of them are from South America, another is from India. They're at different stages of life, ranging from twenty to forty, but they have a shared kindness that has connected us closely this semester. They grab the gift bags and bring them to me before I can even take off my coat.

The first gift is a little boy's outfit—a blue onesie with a bowtie and a plaid shirt to go over it. Before I can even start blubbering, Anna talks about Geo as if he is really going to be born. She says, "I wanted to get clothes that he can wear when he is a couple months old."

And so the conversation goes: each woman exclaiming how they can't wait to meet my little boy, how I have to bring him in after he's born so they can all meet him. They talk about Geo in such concrete terms that I believe them—that I will deliver him, that he will be healthy enough to wear this outfit and meet my students.

I open the other two gifts. Scarves. Beautiful, intricately woven scarves. One of them has blue thread that looks iridescent. It reminds me of the blue wool in my Guatemala shawl, and it's nearly as thick. I feel instantly drawn to it.

The students read from the magazine they created of their best stories and pride warms my soul. At the end, they thank me over and over for all of my help. They stand in line to hug me. I leave feeling that tickle of gratification in my core that makes me love teaching so much.

Once I'm in my car, two words form in my brain: *Fuck it.*

I am choosing denial. I am choosing to pretend that my baby is healthy. I will go maternity clothes shopping with Mom and Dana today. We will pick out a Christmas tree and hang Geo's stocking. We will talk about Geo as if he has the brightest of futures, as if, next year, at Christmas, I will show him the monkey ornament Mom got him, and say, "Grandma got this for you last year when you were still in my belly."

Yes, today I will behave as if Geo is guaranteed to live forever.

On my ride home, I fish through the bags in my passenger seat until my hand grasps the thick fabric of the blue scarf. Though there is ice on my windshield, I try to conjure the warm evening in Guatemala almost a year ago when I teared up from happiness while sitting on the deck overlooking Lake

Atitlan. How content I felt, surrounded by the lapping lake and kind women. How comforting the moon's light felt on my face.

On top of my coral scarf, I wind the blue one.

The weight of them against my chest reassures me.

Later, in Target, Mom looks at me in the fitting room as I show off my bump in a maternity sweater dress. She takes a picture of me and says, "You're going to be a great mom." A worker is making an announcement over the intercom system, and the clerk is throwing plastic hangers into a shopping cart, but, still, Mom's words are clear. She stares at me and her eyes tear.

I shuffle through the other outfits so she won't see my cheeks flushing the same color red as Target's changing room. When I look up, she is still staring, half-smiling, half-crying. And I know that she is wishing with all her might that Geo will survive, that I'll have the opportunity to become a good mother, but she's sad that she won't live close enough to witness it. And I'm feeling the same.

"You're going to be a great mom," she says again, quieter this time.

I repeat her words over and over in my head. I repeat them during the rest of the afternoon and night, and the next morning when we drop Mom and Dana at the airport. I repeat the words until their threads weave together, until their weight on my chest reassures me.

Chapter

28

Though they've tried hard to infuse cheer into the decor, Children's Hospital is the most depressing place a prospective parent can visit. The parking garage is filled with out-of-state plates, proving that desperate parents will travel any distance to help their children. Jamie and I join the mob that migrates from the garage to the hospital entrance and we see them everywhere: sick children—children in wheelchairs and casts, bald cancer-ridden children. I have to look away so that I don't start envisioning Geo amongst them.

Kids with IVs sit on brightly colored benches and point at fish tanks. But no amount of purple paint or animal murals can erase our terror. There is a piano staircase next to the regular staircase, and the healthier children jump from one piano stair to the next, marveling at the way the steps light up and play notes.

Jamie and I climb the regular stairs. We are not in the piano-playing mood.

We know when we're escorted to sit down in a conference room with four doctors that the news isn't good.

It's as simple as this: Geo has distended ureters and kidneys. His urethra is also enlarged. The doctors believe that there might be a flap of skin or some sort of partial blockage in his urethra. Blockage in the urethra means a backflow of urine through the ureters and into the kidneys, which means less urine going out, which means less amniotic fluid, which means not enough pressure on the lungs, which means poor lung development, which means the baby dying in utero, or surgery right after delivery, or a child so troubled with issues that the future is grim.

The head doctor, a tall Asian man with a kidney pin on his white coat, tries to lighten the mood by saying, "But the good news is that we saw Geo empty his bladder during the ultrasound and he has a good amount of amniotic fluid, for now."

He emphasizes the words "for now."

Yes, I think, *but if Geo swallows the fluid and he tries to pee it out and most of it just backflows and gets trapped in his kidneys, then eventually there will be no fluid left, now will there?*

Jamie is silent during the entire hour we spend in the conference room and his cheeks are aflame. He looks as terrified as he did when I was rushed into emergency surgery after my egg retrieval. As the doctors speak, I can see Jamie's zoned eyes refusing to register anything else. Panic has shut him down.

Usually, Jamie is so calm and neutral that I've wondered if anything could emit a strong emotion from him. I've tested him at times, done ridiculous things to make him laugh spontaneously—naked jumping jacks, for instance. During our fights, I've yelled, just to see if he'd yell back. *Just react,* I'd dare him in my thoughts. I've provoked him to joke and shout. But I've never wished for this. I've never wished for us to be in such a sad situation that his mind would collapse from its rage. It's my turn, I realize now. It's my time to return just a pebble of the mound of support he has given me. So, I take charge.

I hold Jamie's hand, ask all the questions.

"Can we do anything to fix it while I'm pregnant?" I ask.

The urologist with the kidney pin, Dr. Li, explains that a shunt can be placed to bypass the blockage in the urethra, but that this sort of invasive in-utero surgery comes with great risk. I ask when the earliest induced delivery might happen if Geo is in danger, and they need to get him out. Twenty-six weeks, they say. The end of my second trimester. Eight weeks from now.

When there is nothing left to discuss, the nurse slides over a blue folder with notes from today's meeting and talking points for our checkup in two weeks. The specialists stand and shake our hands. One of them, a female doctor, is pregnant. As she walks out of the room, I damn her for having what I assume is a healthy baby and a thriving pregnancy. My burning jealousy from our IVF days is back, and it seems it has morphed from sad envy into angry spite.

If we can't be happy, I think, *no one else should be allowed the privilege.*

Still, despite my malice and shock, I am holding it together.

Jamie and I head downstairs, to the cafeteria. Between the drive to the hospital, the waiting, the ultrasound, and the meeting, it's been a five-hour ordeal, and my stomach grumbles with hunger. We get soup and sit down across from each other in the middle of a field of empty tables. The blue folder from the nurse rests next to my bowl of chicken noodle, and Jamie eyes it repeatedly until I slide it into my bag, out of sight.

Jamie brings little spoonfuls of minestrone to his mouth, then abandons it. The redness in his cheeks hasn't subsided. Though hippie affirmations and Buddhist quotes are usually what help me off the ledge, Jamie is a man of logic.

So, I lay out our plan as my thumb traces the Celtic knots on his wedding band. I speak in a firm and assured voice, even if that's not how I'm feeling.

"We are going to come here every two weeks for ultrasounds to look at his fluid. We only have to make it through eight weeks, and then, if need be, Geo can be delivered. He may need surgery, he may need to stay in the NICU. But we and the doctors will do everything in our power to help him survive and live a normal life."

Jamie looks away from me, his face still red, and he says, "But even if Geo does survive, what if his . . ." Jamie gestures toward his groin. "What if his junk is messed up? He won't live a normal life. He'll be made fun of. He won't be able to date. He won't be able to have a family."

I pause, taken aback by how different our fears are. I am thinking in the short term—Geo surviving in utero—while Jamie is thinking in the long term—Geo surviving high school. But, I realize, this isn't much different than our failed embryo transfer last August, how I cried in public at Barnes & Noble and Jamie lost himself in his work. We're both coping with the same bad news, just in different ways.

"OK," I say, "even if that's the case, you'll teach Geo to have the confidence to get through it. You'll be that kind of dad."

I don't know how much Jamie believes me, but he nods. Maybe my brain and body have been through too much to process the worry. Maybe it's not composure I'm feeling, but numbness. I know that the anxiety will creep back into my brain at night, when I lie awake in the dark thinking of the scary information that's in the blue hospital folder, but *for now*, I need to be strong for Jamie, just as he has been so many times for me.

On our way out, I grasp Jamie's hand, and lead him down the piano stairs. The steps light up pink and green and orange beneath our shoes. They play notes of a song to which we don't know the tune.

But we keep stepping nonetheless.

Chapter

29

The genetic counselor announces that Geo does not have trisomy 13, and hope propels us through the holidays. But Geo's hydronephrosis still threatens his survival and my positive thinking wanes as the doctors' visits drag on. It seems like all of January is one big appointment. Between the ultrasounds to check my cervix and the ones to check Geo's kidneys, we are at a different medical office every week. Jamie and I preoccupy ourselves with the logistics: How early do we need to leave work? How long will it take to get into the city during rush hour? We drive to hospitals, park in parking garages, take stairs and elevators to our fate. At each appointment, we wonder if my cervix is too thin, if my amniotic fluid levels are too low.

I lie back on tables and pull up my shirt and technicians spread goop over my skin. They glide wands over my growing bump. We stare at the screen for answers, holding our breath.

We get the same news each time: "Things look the same. For now."

We hear "for now" more than we hear hello or goodbye.

We drive home in silence after each appointment, the sky

already black at five o'clock, and we think about the very clear message the doctors keep communicating to us: Nothing is a guarantee. Things could change at any time.

The blue Children's Hospital folders pile up in my nightstand drawer. I know that a good parent would read the notes and research Geo's condition. Not me. If there's nothing I can do about it, then I don't want to know more than the awful information we've already been presented. But I wonder if I am making the same mistake as I did with IVF. Should I be poring over case studies and seeking second opinions? Could my lack of knowledge be detrimental to Geo's very existence?

A woman's second trimester is supposed to be her best. No morning sickness, more energy. But my brain is constantly preoccupied. I lock my keys in my car. I forget which essay assignment I gave to which class. One thing I do know, at any given minute, is where I am in the countdown to twenty-six weeks—the point when Geo could be delivered and operated on. When people ask how far along I am, my brain automatically responds with, *Four weeks and two days from my third trimester.*

Film reels of hypothetical situations project onto the movie screen of my mind. In one, I don't have enough amniotic fluid and Geo's lungs don't develop and he dies. In another, my cervix gives out and Geo is delivered much too prematurely and he spends his infancy in the NICU. Or he dies. The third is that he develops just fine, but needs surgery right after delivery. Then it's a coin toss—he either survives the surgery. Or he dies.

I don't share these visions with Jamie, and if he has the same nightmares, he doesn't share them with me. Instead, he copes by job searching and interviewing. His boss has recently used up the company savings on his own extracurriculars, and the HR manager confides in Jamie that they might not be able to make payroll and contribute to the employees' health insurance anymore. Jamie scrambles to contact a former employer who happily welcomes Jamie back. Though this means a salary cut, at least he will have job security, and we will have the assurance that his paychecks won't bounce.

At night, Jamie watches comedy shows on repeat—Dave Chappelle, Jim Gaffigan, Nick Swardson. He sits down in his recliner with the lights off and sighs, and I can feel, in that single sigh, the weight of everything that he fears but won't say aloud. When he clicks on the television, he switches off his worry and escapes into a different reality, where his unborn son is not teetering between survival and death. Every now and then, Jamie lets out a truly hardy laugh. When I hear his bellow reverberate upstairs to our bedroom—where I am lying in bed, paralyzed by fear—it makes me smile, if for a moment.

We tell few people besides Mom and Dana about Geo's hydronephrosis. We don't want anyone's sad reactions to make us feel worse. We've learned from all of our IVF hardships that people really have no clue what to say when you share disappointing news with them, and even though all you want them to do is listen and nod and hold your hand, they rarely do. They can't resist relating it to their own troubles or telling you to look on the bright side.

Each time Jamie and I share bad news with others and get poor reactions, I am reminded of times when I, too, reacted the wrong way. I shake my head at the memories, wishing I could go back in time and talk some sense into myself.

When my friend miscarried a few years ago, I met her at a Barnes & Noble café and gave her generic advice, asked her too many questions. I was trying to show that I was concerned, but my clumsiness with the delicate conversation only repelled her, and she had to get up from the table to walk around the store and steady her breathing. The panic on her face was visible, and she ended our coffee date early. She nearly ran to her car. I've been making many silent promises to the universe lately, and one of them is this: *If you let our son live, I will never react badly again. Anytime a friend confides in me, I won't give advice or connect it to my own story. I will simply listen.*

I feel like, during one of my many ultrasounds, the doctors are going to find an extra organ in my abdomen—some tiny bean-shaped thing comprised of my intuition, because I always feel it churning. So often it has made correct predictions, and alerted me of danger, or put me at ease. When I have nightmares and horrible visions about Geo, I consult it, and it responds with a mental embrace that everything will be OK.

I recite affirmations, but I did the same thing during IVF when I drew stick-figure sketches of us holding a baby, and this only resulted in an obsessive love for a child that didn't exist.

So what are we supposed to do?

We simply continue to exist. We wake up, we eat eggs, we drink tea, we go to work, we come home, we pet the dog, we make chicken and asparagus, we sit down at the dinner table, we talk about lighter things, we load the dishwasher, we watch the Food Network, we hug, we go to sleep. We do it all again the next day. We wish for time to pass as quickly as possible so we can make it to the next ultrasound.

Some evenings we talk about our son as if he is a toddler cuddling on the couch with us, some days we avoid his name as if he has already died and his urn rests on the mantle alongside Grandma Kenney's.

Chapter

30

When people notice my protruding belly, they ask a series of questions: *Have you registered for your baby shower yet? Have you started looking at day cares? Have you set up the nursery?* And on it goes. I want to explain that we haven't done these things because we don't know if our baby is going to survive. In fact, we don't know, at this very moment, if Geo is trying to pee and the urine is just backflowing and flooding his kidneys. So, instead, I say, "Not yet."

If tonight's journey to the hospital is any indication of the news we'll receive at the appointment, I'm worried. It takes us almost two hours to get into the city and once we arrive, we circle the packed parking lot for a spot. When we finally enter the hospital, I see a mother pushing her teenage son in a wheelchair. Unlike the other times we've seen these sick children and I've felt sad, tonight I am angry. I'm cursing the heavens. It's the same cliché that everyone wonders, but I'm still thinking it: *Why did the cosmos decide to make this teenager and these children sick?* They've done nothing to deserve this. How different my own teen years were from the boy in the wheelchair's. I ran track. I went to parties. My biggest concern was whether Mom would catch me sneaking in after curfew. Now I wonder what sort of future Geo will have.

Will he have a future at all?

As we sit in the waiting room, I stew about what we might see on the ultrasound screen. Jamie and I sit holding hands, looking at the other couples, and I think, *We shouldn't be here.* None of us should. Maybe we've done something to deserve life's payback, but if illness is fate's form of punishment, then punish us, not our babies. I'm pissed, and I tell the universe this. Mentally, I say, *Enough. ENOUGH. If the ultrasound shows that things have gotten worse, then I'll* . . . but I can't finish my threat. And that's the most infuriating part of all of this. There is not a single thing I can do about any of it.

Finally, our name is called, and we're led to the dark ultrasound room. We've been here so often that we can translate the medical verbiage now. If the tech says distended or dilated, it's cause for concern. One word, however, that we are unfamiliar with is *better.* But as the tech rolls the wand and points at the screen, that's what she says.

"Things look better."

And we can see it, just by looking.

Geo's amniotic fluid has grown to a healthy lake around his body. His right kidney looks smaller.

"The doctor will confirm everything," the tech says. "But this is a definite improvement."

The size of the conference room we are led to reflects the positive news. There is no long table. Dr. Li isn't flocked by four other doctors. It's just him and the nurse in a tiny meeting room with two chairs and a kidney chart.

"His kidneys both still have a little fluid," Dr. Li says. "But, for now, it's nothing too concerning."

Jamie and I look at each other in disbelief.

"Really?" I ask, unable to trust his optimistic tone.

He nods and smiles.

This time, I open the blue folder as soon as the nurse gives it to us. Her notes describe the decreased kidney fluid and the reduced distention in the ureters. Even her handwriting looks cheerful.

Of course things could change at any moment. We still need to keep coming back for checkups, and make it to twenty-six weeks, and early delivery is far from ideal, and Geo might still need to have surgery, but this small bit of progress is the first encouraging news that Jamie and I have heard in a long time, and we're holding on to it as tightly as we hold each other's hands upon leaving the conference room.

On our way out, I skip down the piano stairs, or as close to skipping as any pregnant woman can manage. We drive home from the appointment smiling and linking fingers over the center console.

Jamie says, "I wonder if Geo's dick skin shrunk or something."

"Dick skin?" I ask, grinning. It sounds like the funniest word pairing I've ever heard. It is so nice to say something besides megalourethra.

"Dick skin," we say together. "Dick skin. Dick skin. Dick skin."

We laugh and laugh until my belly shakes and our stress vibrates away.

The countdown continues. I have two weeks, then one week, and then, I can hardly believe it, but I finally make it to twenty-six weeks.

Depending on Geo's amniotic fluid, I could be induced at any moment, but because we've been operating on "maybe" for so long, I have to repeat "will" to myself over and over so that I actually believe Geo *will* be born. It's not an easy thing to do. My perspective on life is different now. Reassuring news feels temporary and conditional. I'm afraid to settle into it, for fear I'll soon be ejected out of its comforts.

But just as we continued on with life after receiving bad news, we play our roles now, too, and are even able to celebrate.

I plan a surprise weekend trip to one of Jamie's favorite places: North Conway, New Hampshire. We get to relax for the first time in a long time. We stay at a hotel and I lounge in the pool, watching little kids splash in the kiddie sprinkler, imagining Geo among them. Will he be like the energetic boy who runs under the waterfall or will he be like the quiet toddler who sits on the stairs dipping his feet into the water?

For dinner, we go into the village center. Jamie loves the quaint downtown with its little restaurants and funky general store. It's a two-level shop with old wood floors and every item you could imagine, from penny candy to quilts. There, Jamie picks out a night-light for Geo's nursery that's shaped like a rustic New Hampshire cabin we once stayed in. I choose little wooden letters with wheels and magnets that connect into a train. As people in thick coats and snow boots enter the warm store, I stand still, holding the letters in my hand—G E O.

I stare at them in wonder.

How long we've ached for you, I think, *and soon we will welcome you into this world.*

"You're already such a good mama," Jamie says, but I don't believe him.

Yet he's been catching me doing things lately, like when I write in the journal that I keep for Geo. I sing "You Are My Sunshine" to my belly as I lie in bed and trace Geo's foot near my rib cage. I devour parenting books and give Jamie the synopses. I research cribs and child-care centers. I sit in Geo's nursery and visualize him in my arms as I hum to my stomach.

"See," Jamie says, standing in the doorway. The hallway light outlines his form.

"What?" I ask, a little embarrassed.

"You're a good mama," he says, and he leans down to kiss me. *Could it be?* I think. *Is it possible?* I am sure I will have many awful parenting blunders, but imagine if I'm actually capable of having moments, every now and then, when I am the mother that I visualized two years ago when we sat in the Lincoln Park cupcake shop and decided to start trying for kids?

Maybe IVF and Geo's hydronephrosis taught me something. Maybe it taught me both grief and gratitude. Maybe it even taught me how to pause.

Maybe, all along, it's been teaching me about motherhood.

Chapter

31

had a revelation recently.

It's shocking that it has taken me this long to realize it, but here it is:

I'm going to have to *deliver* this baby. As in, he is going to have to come OUT of me. FROM my nether regions.

I ask veteran moms about their birth experiences, and most of their stories are unnerving: *My OB was never in the room. A crabby nurse did most of the labor coaching. C-section. C-section. C-section.*

Jamie and I watch the documentary *The Business of Being Born*, and our eyes are further opened.

As the title suggests, the film reveals that many OBs think of birth as a business. In order to save time and make more money, they unnecessarily push Pitocin and epidurals and C-sections.

There is one thing I know for sure after my post-egg-retrieval surgery. I do NOT want to be cut open again.

The film promotes the use of doulas, and Jamie's cousin, Amy, who sent me the email saying, "You will have a baby, of this much I'm sure," is a labor coach. A modern hippie who lives in western Massachusetts, Amy water-birthed all three of her children at home with the help of a midwife. She is one of the most chill people I have ever met.

When I ask, she happily agrees to be our doula, and I can already envision her sitting with me, rubbing my arm, whispering encouraging words. I feel so proud of Jamie and me for taking control over the type of birthing experience we'd like to have.

"What are your hopes for the delivery?" Amy asks us one Sunday as we talk to her on speakerphone.

"I want a natural birth," I say.

I'm not saying this because I'm trying to prove my strength. I'm saying this because the alternative is unthinkable.

Flashes of my emergency surgery continue to haunt me, and I can still feel the soreness of my severed abdomen, forbidding me to sit up. I remember the terror that the night brought, how it convinced me that I'd die in my sleep. How can I nurture a newborn if I can't even move? How can I give him a healthy start if I am anxiety-ridden?

"What are your fears?" Amy asks.

"I'm afraid of having a C-section," I say, "because of . . . because of what I went through before."

And, I think. And . . . And I'm afraid of being cut open again. And I'm afraid of having a careless doctor. And I'm afraid of the drugs. And I'm afraid something will go wrong. And I'm afraid of having another scar. And I'm afraid of hemorrhaging . . .

"I'll be there for you," Amy says. "And when you go into labor, and you're afraid, just remember that it's pain with a purpose."

I am not sure how my OB will feel about a doula. My obstetrician is the doctor who diagnosed my hypothyroidism and prolactinoma two years ago, so I feel somewhat loyal to her, but some of our recent appointments have felt rushed. She is more of a traditionalist, so the idea of a labor coach might not go over well.

We've just finished my checkup, and I tell her that I'd like to discuss using a doula during Geo's birth. "Birth," to me, is such a beautiful word, but in this sterile exam room, under these florescent lights, it feels clinical.

"Doulas . . ." she says, choosing her words carefully, "doulas sometimes try to interfere with doctor's recommendations."

"Uh-huh," I say. I don't want to get on her bad side, but I'm going to have a doula, regardless of whether she likes it or not. So, I change the subject. There's a waiting room full of patients in line to see my doctor, and as if on cue, she checks her watch, but I'm not letting her rush me.

"So what happens if I go into labor when you're not in the hospital?" I ask. The paper crinkles under my maternity jeans as I shift uncomfortably.

The doctor says that she's at the hospital three days a week and will try her best to be at the birth.

"What about the four days you aren't there?"

She says that, in that case, one of the other doctors in the practice would deliver Geo.

"How many other doctors are there?" I ask.

"Nine," she says, placing her hand on the door, cuing that I should wrap up the conversation.

Nine?!

My intuition sounds an alarm.

"How do I meet them?" I ask.

"We don't really *do* that," she says.

Do what? I think.

"I can tell you about them," she says, sighing and sitting back down. She crosses her legs, and though I admire a well-dressed woman, her nylons and high heels don't give off the "natural" vibe I'm going for.

She proceeds by giving me a brief profile of each doctor in the practice and explaining how a couple of them like to be "in and out." This, I have learned, is code for "C-section."

By the time I leave her office, my intuition is screaming, *Something's not right here.*

It's that little nudge I get when something's off. The one I got when we sat in our reproductive clinic waiting room listening to our IVF doctor shout into her cellphone about taking her aggression out on the tennis court, and the feeling I got after our egg retrieval when I saw the wary look on the doctor's face before I went home to recover. It's screaming at me now. This time, I'm not going to ignore it.

Though I've been warned against it, the next day, I call one of the other OBs in the practice to meet her. She prefers natural births, and I hope that she'll be my backup if my doctor isn't available. But, in return, I get a phone call from a nurse, scolding me for going against the rules. She reiterates that I am not allowed to meet with the other doctors.

One positive thing that has come out of IVF is this: I'm not putting up with any bullshit anymore—not when it comes to my health, and certainly not when it comes to Geo's. I want to go into the birthing process with as little apprehension as possible, and it's unsettling to know that some "in and out" doctor might deliver our son. If I am going to be reprimanded for wanting to meet the doctors who might deliver our child, then, clearly, this is not the place for me. I need to switch practices. But whom do I choose, and who will take me at this point? I'm due in three months.

Jenn tells me about the midwife group that she goes to, and how they have an open house once a month.

On a cold February night, Jamie and I attend the open

house, and I immediately feel like I'm home. The midwife, Adrian, talks about labor support and avoiding unnecessary interventions. Because these are modern midwives, their patients usually labor in the hospital's Jacuzzi tubs and an OB always stands by on backup.

Unlike our experience with the IVF doctor, I don't feel like I'm being sold. The midwife acknowledges that this type of experience isn't for everyone, and if you want to come on board, great. If not, there's no judgment.

My first appointment is with the veteran midwife, Valaree. Her moves are yogic, every gesture a pose. She sits in the chair and pretzels her limbs as she talks in a singsong manner. She has a gray pixie cut and wears a beautiful blue scarf that she knitted herself. Even the office is different. A lamp gives the room a soft glow.

We talk about my IVF horrors and my delivery wishes for over an hour. She nods and places her hand on my wrist, in a "Yes, go on" sort of manner.

There are only three midwives that do the delivery, she explains. They all encourage natural birth, and I will have rotating appointments so that I meet all of them as well as the backup obstetrician.

And they love doulas.

When I utter "doula" and "midwife" to people, they tend to recoil, imagining me laboring in a straw hut on a dirt floor. They think I'll have to reach down and pull my own baby out of me, and that I'll be given nothing more than an aloe leaf to recover.

"But don't you want to give birth at a hospital?" they ask. "What if you want painkillers?"

"I *will* be delivering at the hospital, and I *can* have drugs," I say, a bit too defensively. "Doulas and midwives just try to support natural birth, that's all."

I can't lie and say that I don't care about other people's judgment, because I do. I guess I just care much less than I used to. I'm following my gut, my instinct. And that's all that matters.

But their fears make me nervous, and I'm reminded of the tragic memoir called *An Exact Replica of a Figment of My Imagination*. The author, Elizabeth McCracken, moves to France during her pregnancy and chooses a midwife to monitor her pregnancy. One day, near her due date, when she feels the baby moving less, she visits the midwife, who uses an audio Doppler rather than a picture ultrasound. The midwife declares that the baby's fine, just sleepy. But sleepy the baby is not. The cord is wrapped around his neck and he dies. The author has to deliver a stillborn son.

The thought makes me fear that in my stubbornness to strive for a natural birth, I'll risk Geo's life.

But that's not going to happen to us, I reason.

We would know if something were wrong.

Wouldn't we?

Chapter

32

I wait for Mom and Dana near baggage claim at T.F. Green airport. When they come down the escalator, they both see my belly at the same time and say, simultaneously, "Holy shit!"

They hurry down the moving stairs, drop their bags, and wrap me in hugs.

Unlike their December trip when they reassured me that I was tiny, now they exclaim at the hugeness of my belly. It's the beginning of April and they're in town for my baby shower.

Mom rubs my stomach and says, "I can't believe it!"

Dana's mouth hangs open, then, hesitantly, she asks, "Can I feel him?"

I guide her hand near my left ribcage, where Geo's foot is, and he kicks back into Dana's palm.

"Crazy!" she says with wide eyes.

As we head outside, where Jamie pulls up, Mom and Dana walk on either side of me, holding my hand.

I am so damn happy to see them.

"You look beautiful," Mom says, rubbing my arm and kissing my cheek. And despite my sweatpants and runny nose, I do feel lovely, linked arm and arm with my sister and my mother.

The next day is our big appointment at Children's Hospital. The pictures of Geo's bladder and kidneys and urethra will reveal if his amniotic fluid levels have lowered over the past few weeks and whether I'll need to be induced.

Even though it's a sunny spring day and I'm optimistic, I can't help but think about how things went the last time that Mom and Dana came for an appointment.

My mind fills with what ifs as the four of us drive into Boston. Just entering the traffic congestion and the packed parking garage of the medical district gets me thinking of all our previous appointments here. Even though our last meeting was great, the doctor's parting words were "For now."

Whether it's intentional or not, Mom and Dana do a great job of keeping me preoccupied. We're early, so we walk around outside, enjoying the sunshine. While Mom chats away, Dana power walks ahead. Even though Dana is only 4'10", she always walks quickly, and today is no different. She keeps having to stop and turn around to wait, smiling at us slowpokes. I'm usually right there with her, matching her pace, but not as of late. Jamie holds my hand and I saunter slowly, trying to ignore my most recent pregnancy perk—shin splints. But I don't care about the pain shooting up my legs. I'll take any ailment in exchange for a good appointment this afternoon.

In the doctor's office, the receptionist informs us that they're behind schedule, so we hang out in the waiting room, laughing and talking. Even though I feel good, there's still a bit of fear that one bit of bad news will ruin not only my baby shower weekend, but our future too. Even if Geo's amniotic fluid is OK, what if his urethra is distended and he has to be operated on postdelivery?

Finally, my name is called and we all head into the ultrasound room.

Once the gel is on, and the screen lights up, all we see are nostrils and lips. We stare, tilting our heads, dumbfounded about Geo's features.

"Are you sure that's my baby?" Jamie jokes, squinting at the screen.

"Those are Nadine's lips for sure," Mom says.

"And whose nose is that?" Dana asks, looking at the wide nostrils.

The whole time we chirp, laughing about Geo's distinct physical features, I'm anxious for the ultrasound specialist to get to his organs.

When she starts moving the wand, I think, *Please. Please.*

I can tell as soon as she zooms in on Geo's bladder and kidneys that they look as healthy as they did last time. But his urethra is a different story. It's so small that I have no clue by looking whether it's healthy or not.

The ultrasound technician feels good about things, but we won't have the final word until we meet with Dr. Li.

So, now, there's more waiting.

We're escorted to the same small conference room as last time. This should be a good sign, but what if the big scary conference room is just occupied and we're still going to get bad news?

The minutes seem like hours. Mom tries her best to keep me talking, but I grow silent with worry and stare at the wall diagram of normal and abnormal kidneys, ureters, and urethras. The drawings show the differences between the two, but they do not show the repercussions—how one side means a healthy existence, and the other means a life in hospitals.

Which side will the doctor point to in Geo's case?

Finally, Dr. Li knocks and enters, with an assistant who will record notes. Dr. Li is smiling, but this doesn't mean anything, as he had the same nervous grin during our first appointment when he discussed the possibility of Geo not surviving in utero. I place my hand on my belly and take a deep breath while Jamie jiggles his knee. Dr. Li motions toward the kidney diagram.

He points to the healthy urethra, and says, "I can't believe I'm saying this, but there's no evidence of the megalourethra at all." Jamie and I exhale with relief. Mom actually gives a little clap. I barely hear anything he says after that, I'm just so elated. Dr. Li mentions something about the left kidney having a little fluid, nothing too serious, and he'll need to see us back here after I deliver, for a checkup.

"Honestly," Dr. Li says, shaking our hands, "this is the best possible news we could have hoped for."

Though I wish my Chicago friends were here, and there won't be an Illinois shower because I'm too afraid to fly while pregnant, I'm so happy to have Mom and Dana and Jenn and Kelly and Tiffany and my teacher friends and our doula at my baby shower. It's another sunny April day, and Judi is hosting the party at her house. Jamie's parents have always dreamt of retiring to their lake house in Maine, and their Massachusetts house sold recently. So they are relocating up north at the end of April, and this is the last gathering in Jamie's childhood home before the move.

Originally, Judi was going to watch Geo during the three days I'm teaching in the fall, but now we need a backup plan. The thought of having no family around terrifies me. I'm jealous of people who have relatives nearby to help raise their children. Should we stay in Massachusetts if Jamie will no longer have family tying us here? In the depths of my analyzing, I secretly fantasize about us moving back to Chicago. But it seems like such an impossible feat to sell our house and find new jobs while raising a newborn. It's not something we can tackle right now, and today I just want to enjoy this long-awaited event.

I open present after present: knitted blankets and a car seat and a monogrammed toy chest. Both Judi and Mom have held on to Jamie's and my baby clothes and memory books. On my belly, I place a yellow outfit that Jamie wore at the hospital when he was born. I cannot believe that there is a baby inside of me that is going to fit into these clothes. Though my bump feels enormous, and we saw Geo kicking away in my uterus yesterday, I still have a hard time accepting that there is a human being inside of me that is going to come out in a month. It's wild. It's even wilder that I am at the same sort of event that used to send me into hysterics—and that this time, it's *my* baby shower.

Judi passes around blank cards for everyone to fill out for Geo's future birthdays, and I'm reminded of the day, after Grandma Kenney died, when I couldn't fill out Lily's card because my jealousy was so debilitating. I watch everyone around me writing messages to Geo, and I take it in. After my emergency surgery and failed IVF cycles and negative pregnancy tests and spotting and scary ultrasounds of enlarged kidneys—after all that—here we are.

Here Geo is.

As a thank you, Jamie and I have crafted letters to Judi and Mom about what we admire most in them. I printed the letters and framed them as keepsakes. At the end of the shower, I thank everyone for coming and announce that I'd like to thank Judi and Mom by reading something to them.

Jamie's letter references fond memories of summers in Maine and how supportive Judi was during his cancer—how she stayed strong for him and how she sat with him the whole time he received his first chemo treatment so that he wouldn't be scared. My letter to Mom mentions all the times she played in the pool with Dana and me, how she made every holiday memorable—hiding plastic eggs on Easter, filling our shoes with candy on St. Nicholas Day. I discuss my admiration for the way she quit work to care for Grandma and Grandpa when they were dying.

Shocked and verklempt, Judi and Mom dab their tears as I hand them the framed letters.

There's so much more that the letters don't say, like, *Thank you for dealing with our anger and jealousy during our journey to create a child.* But I hope that Judi and Mom both know it anyway. And it seems, by the way they hug us after everyone leaves, that they do.

The next day, before we drop Mom and Dana off at the airport, we go to a consignment store to buy some of the things we didn't receive at my shower. In the cramped, crowded store, the four of us make asses out of ourselves trying, unsuccessfully, to set up the Pack 'n Play that's for sale. We laugh and laugh as we hold up poles and fabric, each of us insisting on assembling it a different way. The worker finally has to come over. In one swift motion, she yanks the thing into position.

"We're so screwed," I say, laughing. "How are we supposed to be parents when we can't even set up a Pack 'n Play?"

Jamie laughs and shrugs. "I'm sure we'll get the hang of it."

Next, Jamie tries on baby carriers. When we strap a secondhand BabyBjörn onto him, he starts to dry-heave. "What's that smell?" he asks, gagging again. The front of the carrier is stained with a gigantic spot of baby spit-up. Jamie's eyes start to water, and he pinches his nose, saying, "Get this off of me." Mom and Dana and I laugh and take pictures of him as he frantically loosens the straps. We laugh so hard, in fact, that I pee my pants a little, which makes them laugh harder, which makes me laugh and pee even more.

The image of Mom and Dana smushed into our backseat between a swing and a bouncy seat is hilarious. I turn around to check on them the whole way to the airport. "We're fine," Dana lies, her knees drawn into her chest, the swing mobile hitting her in the face.

When we hug them goodbye at T.F. Green, Mom says, "The next time I see you guys, you'll be parents."

Jamie and I stand, waving, as they roll their suitcases inside.

"We're going to be parents," I repeat, hugging Jamie.

And it seems, in that moment, that all is well in the world.

Chapter

33

The end of the semester means one thing for the college coeds on my campus—minimal clothing. Everywhere I waddle, I see girls in tiny tank tops and dainty sandals. I, on the other hand, am sporting long capris and Sketchers because my liquid-filled legs shouldn't be seen by anyone. I feel like I've retained ten pounds of water in the last week. What I would give to see my ankle bones again.

As I sit and check my email after class on Thursday, I get a message from Jenn's husband, Adam, with a picture of their baby boy, Mateo.

I can't even comprehend how, just three weeks ago, I saw Jenn and her belly at my shower, and now I'm seeing her baby, outside of her body. The fact that this, too, will happen to me just blows my mind. But now the big question is *When will it happen?* If it were up to me, I'd like for it to happen now. I'm full-term, Geo is fully formed, and I am fully swollen, so why not get this show on the road?

Jenn was a week early, and my hope is that maybe I'll be early, too.

I try to stay on top of grading and plan a backup exam, so that, just in case I have to desert my students during finals, I'm ready. My hospital suitcase is packed and resides permanently in my trunk, and I hope that we'll get to use it soon.

The day after Jenn's son is born, we do get to head to the hospital.

But not to meet Mateo.

And not because I'm in labor.

We have to go for an entirely different reason.

Because Geo isn't moving.

It happens Friday night, as I'm lounging on the couch, watching a movie with Jamie. At the end of it, I realize that I haven't felt Geo move the entire time. This happens occasionally when he's napping, so I give a gentle push to the top left part of my belly where his feet usually are. I feel the heel of his foot there, but when I press down, he doesn't push back. So, I jiggle my stomach a little, and press harder this time.

I wait.

But there's no movement.

Even though I'm nervous, I'm still convinced that Geo's sleeping.

Jamie notices me pressing my middle a bit frantically and asks what's up.

"He probably *did* move during the movie," I say, "but I just didn't notice."

"I'm calling the midwife," he says, hopping up from his chair and grabbing his phone.

"Let me try drinking some juice first," I say and reach into the fridge. Whenever I eat sweets, Geo dances, so it could just be that he needs a little sugar.

Jamie turns off the TV and starts pacing the living room. When I'm one sip into my orange juice, he asks, "Do you feel anything?"

"Not yet," I say, taking another sip. "It could take a few minutes."

Jamie searches through his phone contact list, and says, "I really want to call them, just in case."

At midnight, we're in the car, driving eighty miles per hour down the Mass Pike. The highway is the emptiest I've ever seen it.

As I look out the window, I alternate between poking my bump and jiggling it.

Jamie looks over and asks, again, "Do you feel anything?"

I shake my head. Witnessing his nervousness escalates my nervousness.

Is the cord wrapped around Geo's neck? Is something wrong with my placenta? Did Geo simply stop existing? Could it be that I've made it all the way to full-term, only to have a stillborn baby, as Elizabeth McCracken described in her memoir?

We pass my exit to work, and I have the most horrible thought. *What if I have to tell the sad, sad story over and over again to all the teachers and students who've witnessed my pregnancy—that yes I had a son, but he wasn't alive when he came out?*

I think I'm going to vomit.

The radio is off and the car is so silent I can almost hear both our hearts thundering. Jamie rolls down the window to let in the night air, and it's then that I notice the sweat rolling down his forehead.

I press harder into my belly, harder than I have ever pushed before.

Come on, honey, I say, telepathically. *Move for Mama.*

Then, as we take the Newton exit, Geo's foot gently swipes my rib cage.

"I felt something," I tell Jamie, and he exhales so deeply his whole body sinks in the seat.

I don't want to alarm Jamie by saying, "It was faint, though," so I just reach over and rub his hand.

"It's probably a good idea to still get checked out, anyway," I say, and Jamie nods, taking the exit to the hospital.

The nurse sits me in a chair and belts my stomach with a heart rate reader that's hooked up to a monitor. Then, she hands me a cup of sugary liquid and tells me to drink it and wait.

Jamie and I watch the screen quietly, and I fear a flat line, but, right away, there are peaks and valleys.

The nurse says that this is a good sign, but that Geo has to maintain a certain number of beats per minute for an extended period of time.

She stands near the monitor and makes small talk with us, and I know she's trying to distract us from the question that's circling our brains: *What's wrong with our baby?*

"Have you had a tour with us yet?" she asks.

"Not yet," I say, not wanting to explain that we were going to do a tour, but then we found out about Geo's complications, and we couldn't stand the possibility of visiting a maternity ward I might never deliver at.

My belly moves, and Geo's kicks grow more rapid. They're getting stronger, but I'm afraid to look at the monitor.

The nurse nods and asks about Geo's due date.

"He's due in a couple weeks," Jamie says, anxiously tapping his foot against his chair. I know that he is thinking what I'm thinking. *Just tell us everything is OK.*

The nurse asks how I've been feeling, and I tell her I'm not sleeping much these days.

"It's just your body's way of preparing you for when the baby's here and you're waking up every two hours to nurse him," she jokes.

"Great," I say, trying to force a laugh.

Finally she glances over at the screen and my eyes follow hers.

On the monitor, I see the most miraculous mountain range of Geo's heartbeats. But the peaks are so high that I half-joke about the sugar giving him diabetes.

"He's fine," the nurse says. "You're all set."

"He's really OK?" I ask as she unstraps the monitor from my belly.

"He's doing great. He was probably just sleeping," she says as she gives me a handout on tracking fetal kick counts. "Just pay attention to his movements until your due date. But everything looks perfect. You're good to go."

Then she adds, "Unless you want a tour."

I look over at Jamie, and he smiles.

We both say sure.

As I grab my purse and we follow her down the hall, I'm still flabbergasted that the night started with us thinking the worst, and now, at two in the morning, the nurse is taking us around for our own private tour of the maternity ward. I can't even fathom that behind one of these doors, Jenn and Adam are holding their son, and that soon enough, we'll be holding ours.

Chapter

34

t seems as if Geo wants to stay in my belly forever. In yoga class on my due date, the other yogis fear him crowning while I'm in downward dog, but I assure them that he shows no signs of coming out. He'll be a college student with a five-o'clock shadow, playing video games in my womb.

Then, that night, the faintest of period-like cramps spreads through my middle as I'm nuzzling into my blankets on the couch and watching a movie. I stiffen and glance over at Jamie who sits in his recliner, unknowing. I've heard about false labor's erratic nature, so I decide not to tell him unless I feel another one soon.

The clock on the DVD player reads 8:50, and exactly ten minutes later, another cramp comes. *This is it!* I think. *This is it! This is it! This is it!* I can't believe that after all my stressing, Geo has sent me into labor exactly on his due date.

The lantern lights that hang from our curtain rod illumi-nate Jamie's face as I look over at him and contemplate how to present the news.

"I think I just had two contractions," I say, grinning.

"Really?" he asks with a shocked smile. He pauses for a

moment before he gets out of his chair, gathering himself the way he does when he is cooking a complex meal or calming a distressed client: with total controlled focus.

He switches on his labor-tracking app, and we call Amy. She says that if I'm able to lie down through the contractions, I'm still in very early labor. We planned to go to a hotel in Newton because we live an hour from the hospital and I don't want to be contracting in a vehicle during rush hour, but Amy says that since it's a slow-traffic Sunday night, we should just relax and rest for now.

I want Jamie to turn off the movie, play some soft music, snuggle on the couch, and caress me.

Instead, he loads the dishwasher and empties the trash.

"What are you doing?" I call from the couch.

"Getting everything ready," he says. "We don't know how long we'll be gone. I don't want the house to smell like garbage."

His task-mindedness shouldn't surprise me, but what about my romantic labor fantasy?

"Come here," I say.

"I have to get Tess's food ready," he calls back from the kitchen.

There's no use sitting alone, so I shuffle to the fridge and pack a snack bag for the hospital. Another contraction hits—stronger this time—while I'm filling my water bottle.

In the bathroom, I lose my mucus plug, then, when I'm flushing the toilet, I contract again. This one gives me pause. I'm not so sure I could have lain down through it. Jamie marks it in his app timer.

"They're coming regularly," he says. "Ten minutes apart."

Jamie sets me up in our room with LED candles and music, then grabs his towel for a quick shower. On the bed, Tessa coils into a dog-donut and I curl around her. When the next contraction comes, it forces me from a supine position into a tabletop pose. I arrange pillows in a mound before me, and when the next one comes, I hug them and bear down into child's pose. Tessa, my interim doula, stands up and licks my face. The labor app shows that my contractions are surging every eight to nine minutes.

When Jamie dresses and lies down in bed, I lumber over to his side and breathe in his Dove soap skin. He pulls me into his arms and kisses the back of my neck. It's so soothing in the dark, with John Butler Trio playing over the speakers, but then I feel the storm of pain rumbling closer, and I must roll over to get into my hunched position. My muscles tighten, as if my entire abdomen is encased in hard plaster. The cramp spreads from my front to my back, building in intensity—a hand grabbing my insides and balling them into a hard fist, and then releasing slowly. Between each contraction, my body returns to normal, and I burrow back into Jamie's embrace. Before long, his snores reverberate through the air.

"Are you seriously sleeping right now?" I ask while nudging him with my elbow.

Eyes still closed, he murmurs, "I'm sorry, Nader, it's almost midnight. I'm tired."

I look around the dark room for the glowing clock, and see that he's right about the time. *How did three hours pass so quickly?* I wonder.

When the next wave comes on strong, my pillows no longer suffice for gripping. I ask Jamie to blow up my yoga ball and we both head downstairs.

Two invisible vises clamp down and pull the bones of my sacrum apart, threatening to crack my pelvis and hips. Now I know what all the books meant when they stated I'd "feel" the labor in my lower back. I reach for anything to brace against and grab the top of the dishwasher.

Eight minutes later, I grasp onto the dining room table for

support. Sounds emerge from my lips that I have never uttered before—groans and ohms melding together.

"We should go to the hotel," I tell Jamie through gritted teeth.

"Are you sure?" he asks, and I nod, unable to speak.

The highway is empty and dark, just as it was two weeks ago when we drove to the hospital after I couldn't feel Geo moving. I have to unbuckle and spin around in my seat every eight minutes. "Spin" is actually the wrong word, because it's more of a heaving of body weight while trying not to knock the gearshift with my knee. I press my nose to the headrest, hug the back of the seat, and squeeze every muscle, groan-ohming all the while. We drive through the tolls, and I see the E-ZPass signs shrink smaller in the back window, and I hope that the delivery will be an easy passing, too.

Jamie pulls up to the entrance of the Crowne Plaza, and I wait in the car for fifteen excruciating minutes, during which time I have two more contractions. We are afraid that the staff will see me moaning and not allow us to check in, but when Jamie comes to get me and our stuff, there's no way to avoid going through the main entrance.

As I walk through the automatic doors with my giant blue yoga ball, I know they've got to be on to us. Any second now, they're going to tap my shoulder and say, *Excuse me, you can't stay here. I'm sorry, but we don't want your amniotic fluid on our nice clean sheets.* And who could blame them?

In the elevator, two stoned twentysomethings munch on Doritos and look from Jamie, to me, to my belly, to my big blue yoga ball, and back again. It's 1:00 a.m. now, and I know they're thinking that it's either a weird time to aerobicize, or that we are off to a kinky sex-capade.

A half an hour later, Amy knocks on our door. Her presence is instantly soothing. She encourages us to turn off the glaring hall light, and we listen to music in the dark. Over the last few weeks, Jamie's been compiling this playlist, which he calls Geo's Birth Mix, and his song choices are like new presents I get to open one after the other. Lindsey Buckingham and Dave Matthews and Sarah McLachlan and Ray LaMontagne lull me into a languid state as Jamie strokes my arm and Amy rubs sage and lavender oils on my ankles.

At around 3:00 a.m., Amy urges us to get some rest. She lies on the couch, and Jamie and I get into bed, but every seven minutes, I have to hop up and hug my yoga ball.

"OK, one's starting," I say again and again and Amy dutifully clicks the button on the labor app while I groan and ohm. My back feels like a package that someone repeatedly slices with an X-Acto knife, separates with a yank, and digs around inside of.

When the sun rises and filters in through the curtains, I too feel a shift. I'm afraid to stay in the hotel any longer. The contractions are stronger and closer together. Although the magic number is five minutes apart and mine are six, I know that I have entered the transition into very active labor. If we don't leave soon, I'll be forced to deliver our son in this very room.

As we pull up to the ER, I realize that our greatest hurdle is not behind us. It's right in front of us: the hospital—the very place that houses all of my fears. Though we chose this particular facility because it is NOT the same one I went to after almost bleeding to death, it is the same hospital where we received the horrible news about Geo's kidneys.

The large windows and soothing décor do nothing to conceal its true nature. A hospital is a hospital—every needle and scalpel holds the possibility of harm. And yet, as I drop my bag and contract just a foot from the entrance, what choice do I have?

So, I step through the sliding doors and surrender.

Chapter

35

am eight centimeters dilated upon arrival.
Though I am in the most vulnerable of positions—
feet in stirrups, a midwife's hand up my insides—I feel victorious. This is the biggest confidence boost I've ever received.
I am just two centimeters away from delivering. I am the
most badass woman who ever lived. The hospital no longer
seems like a house of torment. It is the place where I am going to deliver our son. I am going to deliver him soon, and I
am going to deliver him naturally.

Jamie smiles and kisses my forehead.

"You're so close," Amy says in that wonderfully nurturing
tone that made us pick her as our doula.

The midwife, Esther, throws away her latex gloves and
tells me I can put my pants back on so we can transfer from
this check-in station to my hospital room.

And to the nurse, Esther says, "This is definitely going to
happen before your shift is over."

My labor and delivery suite is a serene palace. Sun spills
through the large windows onto the wood floors. The Jacuzzi
tub beckons me, and I immediately change so I can get in. Amy
laughs when she sees my bedazzled bikini.

"I look like some kind of knocked-up Malibu Beach Barbie," I say, pointing to the rhinestones on my triangle top. When I chose clothes for my hospital bag a month ago, I didn't anticipate how ridiculous my spring break-style two-piece would look on either side of my enormous middle.

Jamie helps me into the tub while Esther places LED candles around the bathroom. The jets massage my lower back and the warm currents console me as Jamie kneels next to the whirlpool, scooping water with his hands and pouring it onto my belly. "How are you feeling?" Amy asks from her perch on the ledge of the tub.

"My contractions are lighter," I say, slipping deeper under the suds until my stomach is a small protruding island.

"Your body knows you need a break," Amy says.

I shower and step into a loose sundress. It's cotton and comfortable and allows easy access to my nether regions. Best of all, it is *not* a hospital gown. For the first time, medically, I'm making the decisions. I chose the hospital, the midwife group, the doula, the tub room, the outfit. Finally, I am in charge of my hospital experience. I nod to myself, indicating that I'm ready for the labor finale, and, as if igniting the wick, a contraction firecrackers through my back. *It's pain with a purpose,* I think as I reach for my yoga ball. *It's going to bring us one step closer to meeting our son.*

Jamie and Amy are a seamless stream of support. Jamie mops my wet hair out of my eyes, and just when I feel that my lower back will crack open, Amy presses her full body weight through her palms and onto my sacrum, applying amazing counterpressure.

As the pain intensifies, I feel as if I have sipped champagne. Time and people become hazy. I see everything through a gauzy curtain. Hands press against my back, a voice whispers into my ear, "You're doing a great job," fingers rub my arm, ice chips slip into my mouth, limbs lift me from my yoga ball to a lunged position then a squat then back to the ball, a nurse shift ends, a new one begins. Meanwhile, the glow of the morning sun becomes the pink of a sunset. I contract and contract and contract.

Because I take each contraction as it comes, and because I know labor can last a while, I don't think to ask why twelve hours have passed and I still haven't delivered Geo. Finally, Esther checks my dilation and calls out nine centimeters. I expected ten, and I frown. How did it take me an entire day to dilate just one more centimeter? Esther breaks my water, and I contract some more. When Esther leaves and Valaree takes her place, I say that I have the urge to push, even though I really don't feel that instinctual shift that everybody talks about. Regardless, I decide that it's got to be time for this baby to come out.

The nurses strap the fetal monitor around my middle like a belt. Geo's steady heartbeat thumps through a speaker. My brain chants, *My son, my son, my son, I'll meet you very soon, my son.* I lean back on the bed, my feet pressing against the squat bar. Then I take a deep breath and clench down.

I push and push until it seems like my eyeballs will pop out, and I can actually feel the capillaries near the bridge of my nose breaking, but no baby comes out. Someone says, "Push like you're pooping," and I do exactly that. I poop, but no baby comes out. I push till my face turns purple, but no baby comes out.

Over my knees, I see the nurses glancing at each other. One mentions Pitocin and an epidural. She presents a clipboard of forms for me to sign, and Amy shoots her a dirty look. The backup OB enters the room. He pats my knee and says, ever so softly, that a C-section might be in my future.

I cry and cry and say, "Let me push." But when I do, the

fetal heart monitor's steady beats slow almost to a halt. The nurses glance at each other again.

They order me to take off my cotton dress and put on a johnny. That's when time morphs. There is no dreamy drunk haze anymore. Time is now on crack: an epidural needle in my back and "Push, Push, Push" and the fetal monitor going almost flat and "C-section now" and me on the gurney being rushed down the hallway.

And all I can think is, *The last time I was rushed into surgery, I almost died.*

But now "I" is us.

Don't let us die.

Don't let us die.

Don't.

Let.

Us.

Die.

Chapter

36

A blue curtain bisects me. There's the test of the scalpel and there's the doctor saying *Can you feel this?* and me saying *Yes* and the doctor saying *More meds!* and then the slicing of my abdomen and me shouting in pain, *I can feel it oh my god I can feel it!* and the doctor pulling and tugging my abdomen and skin tearing and me saying *I can feel it I can feel it!* and me crying and asking *Why can I feel it!?* and the doctor saying *I can't get in there, her damn pelvis is too small* and a body lying across my abdomen and hands in my body and a final pull and the doctor saying *He's out!* and silence.

The doctor unraveling the cord from our son's neck and silence.

And more unraveling and more silence.

Geo's blue face and silence.

And silence.

Silence.

Chapter

37

A nd then the most blissful cry.

PART IV

Chapter

38

The card on Geo's plastic crib reads:

George James Johnstone V
Six pounds 12 oz 20½ inches. May 20, 2013, 7:12 p.m.

But he doesn't spend much time in the crib. The morning after Geo is delivered, we lie skin to skin, and I graze my lips over the light fuzz of his hair. My eyes flutter, content. A force field of oxytocin radiates from my pores, and I'm riding high. Our sun-filled recovery room is heaven. From our iPod, Geo's mix plays soothing melodies. Jamie and I kiss and smile like someone pressed the rewind button back seven years. We're giddier than when we first met.

When I need to get my vitals checked, Jamie readies himself for skin-to-skin time by unbuttoning his shirt, and I pass Geo to him. There is nothing in this world more endearing than seeing my brawny husband cradling Geo with the gentlest of hands and placing our son's tiny body onto his broad chest.

Every minute in our cheery hospital room feels like an all-inclusive vacation—kind nurses coo at our little boy, room service delivers steaming omelets every morning, Jamie feeds me bits of egg as I nurse Geo.

When Geo is hungry, he roots around on anyone that happens to be holding him. He bobs his face until he finds something to suck on. Sometimes, his mouth gets a hold of Jamie's nose and we laugh as Geo sucks away, frustrated that it isn't producing milk.

Those pristine moments with our son that I imagined so many years ago are here now. I lie in bed staring at Geo for hours. Everything feels like a miracle. He moves his arm, and we exclaim that he's waving at us. He pees, and we marvel that his kidneys and bladder are functioning properly. Geo's skin is still a little jaundice-yellow and he has scratches on his cheek from his nails, but it doesn't matter. To us, he is absolute perfection.

My body tingles with love for Jamie. We smooch and embrace any chance we get. I can feel it—that we are dazzled with each other for getting through the labor and the birth, for surviving and thriving, for creating a human being, for taking care of our son with such tenderness. I want to bottle this deep desire—the buzzing love we feel for each other because we've been through something big together. I know that, with a newborn, there are hard times ahead. How easy it would be if, during those future hardships, I could just dab a bit of this potion on my neck and let it ward off the negativity.

The last time I was operated on, I unwrapped my bandage to find stitches that stretched half the length of my midsection. *What sort of carving experiment might my abdomen resemble now?* I wonder. But when the nurse removes the gauze, my incision is much smaller than I imagined. The way it curves, perpendicular at the base of my previous scar, forms an anchor shape. *An anchor,* I think, *I can deal with that. There's got to be some symbolism in that.* And because I've already been through abdominal surgery, I know how to handle the recovery this time around—get out of bed, walk around the ward, avoid the Percocets, keep on the stool softener, ask for gas-relief pills.

A few people stop in to congratulate us: Jamie's parents, Josh and Ciara and Lily, Mikey and Kelly. When they leave, the room feels empty. I wish my family and friends could be here. In my fantasies, I imagine them, my village—Mom and Dana and Marie and Jenny and Katy and Courtney and Sarah and Theresa—marveling over Geo's cuteness. Thank god Mom and Dana are flying in soon. When I FaceTime with them, I point to the screen and tell Geo that we're speaking to his grandma and his auntie. But these conversations make me sad, too. Minus a yearly visit, this will be his only knowledge of my family—as faces on a screen.

At night, the loneliness and anxiety settles over me, as it did after my egg retrieval emergency surgery, when the darkness would consume me, and I'd dread my inevitable death. But now it's not my own death I'm worried about, it's Geo's. During our nights on the postnatal floor, Jamie and I care for Geo in shifts. As Jamie sleeps in the dark room, I crave daylight and worry about postpartum depression. I pace the tiny hospital room with our swaddled bundle in my arms, wondering if, even though Geo's peeing normally, there might still be a problem with his kidneys that we can't see. His follow-up appointment with Dr. Li is in a couple weeks, but that feels like a long ways away. What if Geo suffers silently in the meantime or gets seriously sick? The more I pace, the more I worry I'll trip on a cord and send Geo flying through the air. The thought of him crashing on the ground forces me into my seat, which only makes me feel more trapped. I'm jumpy and my breathing grows rapid.

How, I wonder, *am I going to care for Geo when Jamie goes back to work if I can't even make it through a couple hours alone without spazzing out?*

In some countries, family members move into the new parents' home and the new mother's only job is to nurse the baby and rest. But this will not be our reality. Our reality is that we will go home to an empty house with no help. The nights here are just a glimpse of what our future will look like once we leave the hospital and visitors stop coming. It's terrifying.

At around 3:00 a.m., the light of the hall contrasts with our dark room and the nurse's silhouette appears in our doorway. She wheels in a blood pressure machine and says, "Hmmm" when she reads my levels. "It's a bit high," she explains. "We'll have to keep an eye on it."

Finally, at 4:00 a.m., with Jamie still sleeping, I seek help. I roll Geo's portable crib to the nursery at the end of the hall. Geo is wearing a soft yellow hat that Jamie's mom knit for him. The nurses take Geo's crib, and through the big observation windows, I can see his bright cap getting farther and farther away. He's just a couple days old and already I feel the tug of motherly guilt, but his plastic crib joins many others, reassuring me that the other mothers on the floor need a break, just as I do.

Though I want, more than anything, to sleep, I can't. So I walk around the hall. I pass the nurses' station, the kitchenette, the elevators, the other patients' rooms, and our room that emits Jamie's snores. I pass the nursery and spot Geo's yellow hat. He's sleeping peacefully. When I feel the pull of pain on the left corner of my incision, I know it's time to stop and reward myself with a treat: a peanut butter and jelly sandwich from the kitchenette. The pantry is filled with juice and instant coffee and graham crackers and saltines and bread and jelly. I haven't had sugary Smuckers in so long. Each sticky bite of my sandwich transports me to lazy summer days at Grandma's house, reading Sweet Valley Twins novels while she watched *Oprah*. Her PB&Js were always the best—gobs of Peter Pan peanut butter and strawberry jelly oozing out the sides when I squeezed the soft bread slices together.

During each of the remaining evenings at the hospital, this becomes my nightly routine—walks and sandwiches—the only things that will ease my anxiety and my longing for my family.

Chapter

39

When Mom and Dana arrive two days after we're discharged from the hospital, Mom is a power-house. She does our laundry and fills my water bottle. As thirsty as I've always been, I've never truly under-stood the definition of "parched" until now. Nursing-thirst strikes every time I expose my breast to feed Geo. It's as if he is literally siphoning the liquid from my cells. And the hunger—my god, the hunger. I'm starving at all times. My metabolism is so revved, I wake up each morning drenched in sweat. The energy expended to produce Geo's milk is like that of aerobi-cizing around the clock. I'm even hungrier than I was during my marathon training days, when I could eat a dozen ice cream sandwiches after a giant lunch.

For the week she's in town, Mom goes to the store each morning and buys pounds of produce—strawberries, grapes, honeydew, and cantaloupe. She sets giant bowls of fruit salad on the coffee table in the living room as I sit in my leather chair and nurse Geo. We are three generations nurturing each other—a mother mothering her daughter, a daughter mother-ing her son.

Geo eats every two hours, and each feed takes around forty-five minutes. It forces my anxious self to just sit and be in the moment. I take advantage of the heat wave and bring Geo to the Adirondack chair in our backyard, letting the sun warm my chest while he nurses. The balmy breeze rustles through the trees and finches land on the branches. It feels like a miraculous cycle—my pores taking in the nourishing rays while Geo feeds from me. I trace every inch of our amazing boy—his feet that are definitely Jamie's, his cheeks that are definitely mine. What a gift he is. How lucky we are.

But as much as I want to live in the splendor of these moments, they also prevent me from doing necessary things like sleeping or going to the bathroom. I'm strapped to a chair, boobs out, for the majority of the day. I haven't slept for longer than a two-hour span, and I'm shaky with delirium. The room shifts when I stand. But what can I do? I am Geo's sole source of nutrients, so if he needs to eat, how can I sleep?

At night, when everyone goes to bed, and I am left to take care of Geo, hot tears stream down to my chin and land on Geo's head that's nestled in my chest. I weep because I'm scared of accidentally dropping him. I weep because I'm so beyond exhausted. I weep because my exhaustion might make me drop him.

So, I pace the house until sunrise, at which point, I pace the neighborhood.

When I come back from a walk one bright morning at around 6:30 a.m., Geo fastened to me in a kangaroo-pouch, Jamie yawns and says, "Don't you think you should take it easy?" But how else do I get through the dawn with a screaming baby while everybody else sleeps?

My sleep deprivation manifests into a sort of mania, like that of a meth addict.

Dana watches over me and takes on chores so that I won't

exert myself. She feeds Tessa and straightens up the living room.

"Relax, Nay," she warns me as I hop out of chairs too quickly or scurry up stairs that a C-section patient shouldn't be traversing. She's right. I know that I just can't keep up this pace. I need help. I need other people to take Geo shifts.

Although most practitioners say to wait a few weeks before pumping breast milk so that the baby doesn't have nipple confusion, I try it out when Geo is a week old. That pump is a godsend. I fill bottles upon bottles, building a supply so that Jamie and Mom and Dana can feed Geo when I need a break. I can leave my post at the chair to shower and make breakfast. I feel like I did after my emergency surgery, when I was able to drive and work again. Now, I flip eggs while smiling and singing, grateful for the extravagance of a perfectly cooked omelet.

So, after days in the house, we finally take Geo for his first trip out into the world. Jamie's back at work, so it's just us girls and Geo. To the strip mall we go. When I order a mocha at the Starbucks café in Barnes & Noble, the worker looks at me, then at my nonexistent belly, and says, "Wait a minute. Something's different."

"That's my son, and my mom, and my sister, over there," I tell her, pointing to the very same spot where I've sat alone almost every Saturday since moving to Massachusetts, trying to self-soothe with caffeine and word documents.

And in that moment, I have a revelation: I sat alone at the café all those times and tuned into Pandora so that I didn't have to think about what I had left behind in Chicago. As I typed away at my nineteenth novel revision during those lonely afternoons, I reasoned that I could not call my friends or Dana or Mom and say, "I miss you." Because I'm the one who chose to leave them. To admit to them that I yearned for their company felt, to me, like some admittance of defeat.

As with any vice, like wine or pills, the solitude was something that made me feel good, but when I was feeling melancholy, I needed it too much, too often. I sat and wrote in my journal so that I didn't have to fess up to Jamie or anyone else that, although I loved parts of my life here, I also missed parts of my old life, too.

Now, nagging dread pulls at my heart. *Mom and Dana are leaving in two days.*

But I can't think about life in Massachusetts without them or going to appointments like Geo's kidney follow-up in two weeks without their emotional support. It's enough to speed my pulse, so I sip my drink and join them. Instead of staring at a computer screen, I baby-talk and tickle Geo. I rub Mom's arm, then Dana's.

"This is so nice," I say. "I've missed you so much."

Chapter
40

We're at Geo's nephrology appointment, and after all of the ultrasounds I underwent while pregnant, now Geo is the one lying on the white paper with a wand sliding across his torso. His newborn body looks too tiny on the table.

He shouldn't be here. No baby should.

He fusses a little. Maybe he doesn't like being held in one spot. Maybe he's realizing that this is simply unfair—an innocent child being poked and prodded for reasons beyond his control. Jamie rubs Geo's foot and says, "It's almost over, buddy." I hold the pacifier in Geo's mouth and *shhh shhh shhh* into his ear. The tech is gentle and puts *Dora the Explorer* on the miniature TV to distract him. As she wipes the gel off of Geo's bare stomach, she tells us that his bladder and kidneys look good, but he still has to undergo another procedure to examine his urethra.

The tech and doctors throw around the term "VCUG," as casually as "LOL," but what it really means is shoving a catheter up Geo's tiny urethra and injecting dye to see if, when he urinates, the liquid goes out the way it should or if it goes back up toward his bladder and kidneys.

As we wait in the lobby, Jamie is quiet. He cradles Geo gently, but his knee bounces an anxious beat.

"You OK, Love?" I ask.

"I just feel so bad for him," Jamie says. "Poor little dude. No guy wants to have something jammed up there."

Geo sucks away on his pacifier, which is the hardest part of all this. He has no idea what's next.

The nurse leads us to a large room with machines and tubes and screens. Unlike the ultrasound room that was warm and dim, here, the lights are bright and the cold air smells sterile. We peel off Geo's white onesie and place him on the table under a large x-ray machine, then prop a bottle in his mouth as the doctor instructs us to hold Geo in place. Even though she explains it delicately, there's no other way to say it: We have to pin our child down and let the doctors shove a giant tube up his tiny penis. Jamie's face is red as he stares at Geo with apologetic eyes.

After explaining the procedure in full, the doctor peels back the skin on Geo's penis and prepares to insert the catheter. Geo sucks away at his bottle, happily, obliviously, until the doctor injects the tube. The force of Geo's screams pushes the bottle out of his mouth. He thrashes, and we have to press our palms against his limbs. Geo uses all of his strength to fight our grasp, and I feel like our resistance will bruise him. We *shhh* and caress him as we hold him down, but he flails and screams. I feel as if I am clasping his arms and allowing someone to beat him up.

It's just awful.

Geo wails and kicks.

After injecting the liquid, the doctor retracts the tube and, over Geo's screams, says, "All done."

Geo must still lie on the table while he urinates, so that they can get x-rays, but at least he won't be in pain anymore.

I'm kissing Geo's forehead and telling him what a good boy he is when I hear the doctor say, "Are you hanging in there, Dad?"

That's when I see that Jamie is crying.

I give Geo his bottle again, and he stops screaming. But as Geo sucks away happily, Jamie's lower lip is still quivering, so I reach over and hug him.

Because Jamie is usually so neutral and always insists he's fine, I've often wondered how all of this—the IVF, Geo's hydronephrosis—has affected him, and I caught a glimpse of it at Children's' Hospital, months ago, when he shut down in the conference room. But now it's fully visible in front of me: the release.

"I just hate seeing him in pain," Jamie says as he wipes his eyes with his T-shirt.

Watching Jamie cry feels as awful as watching Geo writhe in pain, but this is what Jamie has been dealing with for two years as he stood over me in various hospital beds. I reacted to our traumas by fighting and fleeing, but all the while, Jamie has remained still—a silent, sturdy presence. I can't imagine the pressure he must have felt to be my rock, or how often Geo's diagnosis must have triggered Jamie's memories of his own hospital days, battling cancer.

As much as I hated being the one doing the IVF injections and throwing up from morning sickness, I realize now that maybe it was harder for Jamie—having to stand by and watch it all, having to be strong.

Although these days I usually sit in back of Jamie's truck with Geo, on the ride home from the appointment, I sit in front with Jamie. I reach across the center console and stroke his hand, ask him how he's feeling. He doesn't say that he's fine, as he normally would. He spills his fears, and I try my best to be his silent, sturdy presence.

Chapter

41

One day, Geo's doing tummy time; the next he is sitting up. One day we're at the beach; the next we're at the pumpkin patch. This is how the next few months of Geo's life zoom by.

And then, one Sunday in late October, everything screeches to a stop.

It's a beautiful autumn day. We slurp some hearty squash soup at Whole Foods and drive home through the fall foliage. Life is good. But then, that night, nausea jolts me from my sleep. I throw up the way I did when I was pregnant—heaving so much that my head hits the bowl, and I pee my pants. *Please god*, I beg, *don't let me be pregnant.* I calculate back, trying to remember when Jamie and I last had sex. But then, I'm hurling again.

When Jamie wakes up in the morning, he finds me on the floor of the bathroom, curled into a fetal position. He's holding Geo and ready to do the pass-off. It's a non-teaching day, and I'm supposed to be on baby duty.

"Stomach bug?" he asks. "Food poisoning?"

I vomit again and keep the *"Or pregnancy"* possibility to myself.

"Geo has to go to day care," I say. My legs tremble when I stand. I barely make it to the couch before I fall over, dizzy.

What if I'm pregnant? What if I am seriously pregnant? Could it be that after all our IVF struggles, I'm expecting when I don't even want to be? I simply can't grow another human being right now. I can barely take care of myself and Geo and the dog, who's growing more jealous and whiney by the day. The last time I was pregnant, the first trimester nearly destroyed me, and that was when I wasn't raising an infant.

Jamie carries Geo upstairs to change him, but then he runs back down, placing Geo in my lap.

"What's wrong?" I ask. Clearly Jamie doesn't understand how much misery I'm in, or else he wouldn't be leaving Geo on the couch with me.

As an answer, Jamie runs to the bathroom.

He emerges fifteen minutes later, holding his stomach and moaning.

"I think I have food poisoning, too," he says, flopping onto the couch.

Jamie's sickness means Geo is stuck at home, too. Neither one of us can drive the forty-five minutes to his day care near Jamie's work without vomiting or having the hurry-ups. We need family more than ever, but we have no one to watch Geo while we wretch. Jamie and I take turns shakily running to the bathroom while the other moans on the couch and Geo cries in the swing. When carrying Geo to his changing table, my weak arms threaten to drop him. That's when I sink into the couch and surrender.

We. Need. Help.

This is our future, I realize. Unless we move to Maine or Chicago to be near family, this is what every chaotic instance will be like.

Dana must sense the desperation in my voice, because she surprises us and flies in to help out. She has just quit her bank job to become a dog trainer, and she's broke, but she still buys a last-minute plane ticket so that she can spend three days changing diapers for free. I almost cry from happiness when we pick her up at the airport, though I warn her that she may need to change my diaper too. A couple days have passed since Jamie and I got food poisoning, and my body still hasn't bounced back completely.

How much easier life is when there's a third person assisting with bottle and diaper duty. But even better is that we get to hang out and be sisters. We watch bad reality TV and talk, honestly, about life. While lounging on the couch, I rest my head on her shoulder. She jokes that I'm crowding her space, but then she leans her head against mine and leaves it there.

God, how I've missed her.

The morning of her flight back home, we go to the pumpkin patch with Geo. We want to show him the baby squash and Indian corn, but on the hayride, Dana grips her stomach and groans.

"I'm gonna puke," she says. She hangs over the wagon rails as the tractor traverses the bumpy fields. Among the cornrows and apple trees, there's no pull-over spot or port-o-potty in sight.

"Maybe we didn't have food poisoning," I whisper, so as not to alarm the other riders. "Maybe it was a stomach bug."

Great, I think, my guilt building as the tractor struggles up a hill. *There's nothing like rewarding someone for watching your kid than by passing along the bubonic plague.*

The tractor crests and puffs thick clouds of black exhaust

back at us. I cough and wave the fumes away from Geo's face. Then we wend down a trail full of holes and divots. Geo bounces in my arms, and Dana searches anxiously for a way out. With each jolt, I expect Dana's stomach and Geo's tiny body to leap from the wagon.

This was a bad idea.

Finally, the hayride from hell ends, and Dana runs through the gift shop to the port-o-potty. I wait, holding Geo and looking up at the sky that threatens rain. After ten minutes, the plastic door slams, and Dana comes out wiping her mouth. Sweat beads up on her pale forehead.

"How are you going to get on your plane?" I ask as we walk the gravel path to the car.

"I'll be fine," she says.

But fine she's not.

She pukes the whole drive back to our house. I set her up in the guest bedroom with water and medicine. I rub her arm while she squeezes her eyes shut. Tessa rests her head on Dana's calf, trying to soothe her with licks and nuzzles.

But, then, it's time for Dana's flight. She forces herself through security and heads to her gate. Maybe she just wants to get back to her own apartment, or maybe she doesn't want to change another dirty diaper, but, somehow, Dana gets on the plane, clutching a plastic bag that she'll surely puke in the whole eight hundred miles back to Illinois.

I'm sad to see her go, not only because we gave her whatever awful virus we had, but because, after I drop her off, the passenger seat seems empty without her. Back at the house, both Tess and Geo look around, silently asking where Auntie Dana is.

Chapter

42

On the mornings I'm home with Geo, I open all the shades, willing the sunshine to be my companion, to get me through the sometimes monotonous and frustrating days that come with caring for a child alone.

November cloaks the sun with her gray cape and the living room remains just as dark as when the shades were drawn. During these days, loneliness lurks like a shadow.

Two years ago, wasn't I bargaining with the universe that if I could have a baby, I would never complain about anything ever again? And didn't the universe give me what I wanted—a baby—and a healthy one at that? So why am I complaining about my loneliness? For some reason, the desolation seems so much more unnerving with Geo *in* the picture. Shouldn't I feel fuller now that our two-person family has expanded to three? The isolation bugged me before, when I didn't have friends or family to hang out with, but I could distract myself with a Starbucks writing session or a yoga class. The busyness got me through.

I'm reminded of the days after my post–egg retrieval surgery when I came home to recover and the truth of my sadness was so achingly clear. What is it about being in this house with an idle mind that exposes my sorrow so blindingly?

On the days I try to answer work emails and Geo slams his hand on my laptop, on the days when I need to grade student papers and Geo refuses to be put down, on the days when I can't nurse Geo because the stress of being broke has caused my milk supply to dwindle, on those days I slump against the kitchen counter and rub my temples begging the higher power for help. Because I know there is no end to the demand for my love and attention. And I want to give it, but I have no source from which to draw it. I'm empty.

Sometimes I envision her—the apparition that embodies Mom and Dana and all my friends in one nurturing female soul. She pats my hand, takes Geo from me, kisses me on the cheek, and says, "Breathe, get some sleep, read a book, have some wine, paint your toes, see a movie, hug your husband."

But I have to come to terms with the fact that neither this apparition nor marital affection exists. Jamie and I are watchmen on different shifts. When he comes home and watches Geo, I still have dinner and laundry and unpaid bills and student essays awaiting me. I wrestle with time for a half-hour exercise class here, two hours of writing there. But this time doesn't come free. Each minute is accounted for in the tally sheet that has become our lives. Jamie and I must barter for hours. Most of our conversations go something like: "I'll take Geo on Sunday afternoon so you can watch the Pat's game if you can take him on Saturday morning so I can write."

The two of us have barely touched each other in six months.

We need help—*regular* help, *free* help. And I know that if I called Jamie's parents, they'd make the four-hour drive from Maine, but that takes advanced planning. And it's not something they can do on a weekly basis. My fantasies all center around moving to Chicago, where I could call up Mom on a Tuesday morning when I'm plagued by the flu and can't take care of Geo or Dana could watch Geo on a Saturday night so Jamie and I can wear something other than snot-ridden sweats and enjoy dinner without worrying about the baby's sleep schedule. Right now, Geo's only notion of family is the two faces that stare back at him day in and day out. I fear that, soon, Geo will become like Tessa, who stares out the window whining for visitors that never come.

We need a village.

When I moved to Massachusetts, I thought that all you needed in this world was your life partner and your offspring. And this is partly true. Jamie is, without a doubt, my desert-island man. But I don't want to live on a desert island if I don't have to. Desert islands sound more appealing than they actually are—all the hut construction and coconut cracking is your responsibility, and you get so desperate for company that you start mumbling to the sand.

But didn't I move here because I didn't need anyone besides the broad-shouldered man I fell for in Tampa, Florida? Didn't I flee from the very family, the very city that raised me? I reasoned that my family was too loud and obnoxious, my mother too invasive and opinionated, the city too noisy and crowded, my friends too consumed in fast-paced life to enjoy the simple sounds of nature. How can I ask back for the very things I've discarded? And how can I seek their help when, for years, I've prided myself on not needing it?

In Geo's nursery, he and I cuddle in the glider. I wrap him in a thin blanket and give him his pacifier. As we rock forward and back, I read him his usual nap-time book—*The Little Blue Truck*.

In the story, the blue pickup and all of his animal buddies greet each other cheerfully, but when the big dump truck comes through, he's too busy to say hello. Then karma catches up with him.

I point to the pictures and ask, "Do you see how the dump truck gets stuck in the mud?" Geo grabs the board book and turns the page, revealing Little Blue Truck speeding to the rescue. Geo's eyes flutter, but I continue to read on about how the small truck is no match for the mud, either. He gets stuck while trying to push out the dump truck. And so he has to call upon his buddies: the toad, the cow, the chick, the sheep, the goat, the horse, the duck—the same animals that the dump truck had just ignored—to help them.

Geo's eyes droop shut as he breathes deeply, and his body becomes heavy. Before I close the book, I recite the last lines from memory, about the importance of getting help from close friends.

The words catch me off guard, and I can't believe that a damn kids' book is giving me pause, but it is. And I decide, right then, that I need to get over my pride and start seeking some support.

I place Geo in his crib. But before I close his door and tiptoe down the stairs, I turn on his noise machine, to simulate my motherly heart beating in the room with him. Then I call my own mother and ask if she'll help us out with plane tickets so we can visit Chicago for Christmas.

On a cold December morning two weeks before our Chicago trip, Jamie puts on his coat and gathers his keys for work, but when he kisses me goodbye, he pauses.

"What's going on with you?" he asks.

"What do you mean?" I ask, avoiding his eyes.

"Something's up," he says.

I put Geo in his ExerSaucer, and take a deep breath.

It all tumbles from my mouth—the sadness, the yearning

for company. Jamie leads me to the dining room and sits on the leather bench, then pulls me onto his lap.

Our artificial Christmas tree looks anorexic and dull in the light of day. Neither the ceramic snowmen nor fireplace stockings can force merriment.

"I feel like you're just not into me anymore," he says.

"I think I'm really lonely here," I say as I fidget with the zipper on my fleece. "I'm starting to feel resentful, and I'm taking it out on you. I really miss my friends and family, and I think a lot about us moving to Chicago." My voice fades. "But we'd have to sell our house and find jobs. It just seems impossible . . ."

Jamie surprises me by saying, "You know I'm not a city guy, Nader, but I owe you this much."

I look up at him and search his face, asking, *Really?*

He nods and hugs me.

Jamie leaves for work, and I ready Geo's mashed bananas, smiling all the while. The whole idea of moving still seems completely overwhelming, but at least I know Jamie is committed. But then I remember the day, seven years ago, when Jamie told me he'd move to Chicago for me, and how months passed as he job-searched in Illinois, and it was a tough market, and eventually, Jamie just stopped looking in Chicago. One day he called to tell me he'd found a new job—not in Illinois, but in Massachusetts. So, I moved for him. Though it was so long ago, it still stirs up the pain of an unkept promise. I just hope that this time will be different.

Chapter

43

The Chicago that awaits us for our Christmas vacation is a frigid one, and Dana's ailing car barely gets us to the Loop. But the sparkling Hyatt Mag Mile welcomes us thanks to my friend's employee discount. The bellmen treat us like we're stepping out of a limo and not Dana's rusting Cavalier. They whisk our bags onto a cart, and we are instantly lighter, free of our suitcases. As we step into the espresso-whirring wonderment of the Starbucks that adjoins the Hyatt, Dana scoops Geo from his stroller and coos at him. We stand by the revolving glass door laughing about how many times Mom has texted that she's on her way. "You think she's just a little excited to see her grandson?" Jamie asks.

In Chicago we have Auntie Dana and Grandma at the ready, and because of that, I find myself taking slower, fuller breaths and longer, happier exhales. I'm aware of another sort of heaviness we have shed upon arrival—the responsibility of caring for Geo alone.

In our hotel room, I get ready for my girls' night. When I shed my nursing tank and yoga pants for a skirt and satin top, my joy radiates through the room.

"Got a hot date?" Jamie jokes as he shows Mom Geo's latest skill of crawling. And it does feel like a date—a date with my beloved Chicago friends who I haven't seen in almost two years.

When Dana and I drive to the restaurant, I just fear that I won't fit in with my friends anymore. While I've been living the settled life in Massachusetts, they've been enjoying dating and kid-free marriages in the city.

At dinner, the ease of our conversation convinces me that though our lives have changed, our friendships have not. I do feel different, in a way, because I have been through IVF and pregnancy and childbirth, but my friends have also experienced things that I haven't, like the sickness of a sibling and the death of a parent. We have all compiled more losses and joys than we had five and a half years ago, when I moved to Massachusetts.

We catch up and laugh a lot. Dana discusses her dog-walking business plans with Sarah. Jenny talks about her new boyfriend. Courtney distributes Christmas cards featuring her blind adopted dog. Marie gives the waitress a list of food allergies that leaves the poor woman puzzled. Theresa regales us with tales from her most recent trip to Thailand, which included a visit to Bangkok's red-light district.

"So let me get this straight," I say, with scrunched eyebrows, "this girl shoots darts out of her *vagina?*"

We laugh and laugh until all the plates are empty and the wine almost gone. It's Wednesday night, and most of my friends have to go home and wake up early for work. Courtney and Sarah and Dana stay behind to have one more drink with me, and we eventually get on the subject of my desire to move back to Chicago.

"But it's so complicated," I say. "We'd have to sell our house and find new jobs. And I really don't think we can afford anything here."

The girls assure me that even though we'll have to give up

some square-footage, we *can* afford something here, even something with our preferred amenities. Then Courtney adds, "You basically have a three-year window. Once Geo's in school, it's going to be a lot harder to make a move."

Something about this clicks. She is absolutely right. I think that our situation is complicated right now, but once Geo enters kindergarten and makes friends, I'll feel horrible uprooting him. If Jamie and I want to do this, we need to move fast. I understand that if we don't attempt to move soon, it's never going to happen.

I start to persuade myself of all the reasons why right now is actually a good time to relocate. Jamie has already talked about feeling untethered to Massachusetts. His friends have scattered and his parents have moved away. He doesn't love his job. On my end, I have no family in Massachusetts. I can be an English instructor anywhere. The idea of moving morphs from a dream to a possibility, and my brain pulses with the prospect of a future city life.

It's almost midnight when Dana drives me back to the hotel, and Chicago's damp streets are empty, save a couple of drunken wanderers. I'm the sort of happy that you can only get from chatting with your sister and decade-long friends. When I wave goodbye to Dana from the Hyatt entrance, I smile and think, *If I live here, these dinners can be a regular thing.*

But when I tiptoe into the dark hotel room, Jamie's and Geo's soft snores greet me, and I grasp that the larger issue here is not finding an apartment and jobs in Chicago. It is asking Jamie to leave everything he has known for forty years, to disregard his disdain for honking taxis and a concrete landscape. It is plucking Geo from a quiet suburban childhood and dropping him in the middle of an ever-buzzing urban upbringing. It is clear to me, now, that by asking Jamie and Geo to move to the Midwest, I could potentially be destroying our family dynamic and our future. I have to think long and hard about the repercussions of making such a drastic decision. I have to know, with absolutely certainty, that it will be worth it in the end.

Just like with IVF, what if we take the leap and invest our lives in this venture, and it simply fails?

The next day, we visit my old stomping ground in Lincoln Park. We walk down Clark and have Mexican food at my favorite burrito joint, then visit my most beloved LP haunt of all—Molly's Cupcakes.

It's bone-numbing cold and damp outside. The cabs splash slushy snow up onto the curb as they whiz by. Once inside the toasty confines of Molly's, we pull off our gloves and un-loop our scarves, taking refuge at a table near the window that is fogging from the steam of our breaths. The smell of cake batter instantly brings me back. Jamie and I shake our heads at the fact that we sat at this very table three years ago and made the decision to have kids. Now, all those IVF horrors and kidney problems later, here we are with Geo.

I relish in the retro-ness of the bakery. Orb lights hang from the tin-tiled ceiling, and board games rest on the window seat. This homey reprieve from the cold soothes me. I feel as if I have been wrapped in fleece and given a hot cocoa.

After debating over the glass-case display, we indulge in sugar bliss—a Cookie Monster cupcake for me, a chocolate madness for Dana, a red velvet for Mom, and a peanut butter specialty for Jamie. We sit around the circle table, licking icing off our fingers and passing Geo around.

He stands on our thighs and stares unapologetically at the other customers. Openmouthed, he grabs our ears and pulls our faces in, either trying to eat us or kiss us. This is my favorite game to play with him. Imagine loving someone so much you don't just want to kiss them, you want to swallow their whole face. It's as if he's saying, *You fools, kissing is for amateurs. This is how you really show affection.* We laugh and try to turn our heads or pull away, but he always gets our noses, and we squeal as we wipe away the drool. This sends him into fits of giggles.

Geo slaps and bangs on every surface before him—a shoulder, an arm, a table, a plate. *What is this? How does it work?* Mom lets him play with her plastic cup, and Dana makes a surprised face that leaves Geo's dimples permanently indented. I don't know if I've ever seen him this happy. It is so different to be somewhere, anywhere, with family accompanying us. To be surrounded by loved ones warms me so thoroughly that I feel I must be radiating heat. Jamie puts his hand on my lower back and rubs it.

I want to stay here forever—not only in Molly's but also in Chicago.

I want to watch Dana's soccer games and jog along the lake with her. I want Mom to play with Geo whenever she wishes. I want to stop by my friends' apartments on the weekends. I want to walk down a street and see people. My people.

I want my Chicago family back.

Sometimes there are moments in my life when I am aware of a pivotal shift, even as it is happening. It's as if I am standing on the desert earth, and the red clay beneath me begins to crack, and I jump from one side to the other, and the crack gets wider and wider—inches, feet, meters, miles—and I know there is no jumping back over, nor any longing to. Then, that land, that continent, floats away, and I turn my back to it and walk forward into new territory. I felt this way after we lost our two embryos, and I feel it again now. It's time to move on. I know that starting a new life in Chicago is a huge risk. I know that it will forever alter our destiny, but I think—I know—that it is the right choice.

I smile at Jamie and ask him if he'd like to taste my cupcake, but he declines. I know that the very same thing could happen with our move to Chicago. Even though he agreed to the hypothetical idea, if I propose the actual plan, might he say no? Then what?

I think all afternoon about how to ask Jamie to move to Chicago, but the discussion occurs spontaneously the following day as Jamie and I roam around Old Town.

Jamie pushes Geo's stroller and I walk beside him down Wells, pointing out the chocolate shops and the Second City comedy club. It's the area that Jamie originally wanted to live in when he discussed moving here seven years ago. If anyone is going to fall in love with Chicago, it's easiest to do so in Old Town. It has all the perks of the city—tons of cafés and restaurants, parks and public transportation—but it's quaint and tree-lined.

I am about to approach the moving conversation by saying that living in the city does not have to mean living in the chaos of the Loop. It fact, I don't want to live amongst skyscrapers and screaming taxis. City life can actually mean living in a neighborhood like this. But Jamie cuts me to the chase. He points at apartments that look appealing and says, "I wouldn't mind living in a place like that."

I agree with such fervor that he knows I'm serious.

"So this is really going down?" he says.

I nod my head. And that's it. That's the end of the conversation.

That was the easiest life decision we've ever made, I think.

But that night, Jamie's mood morphs. He criticizes the congested traffic and the crowds on Michigan Avenue along with the dry hotel air and the stiff bed. He wants familiar things like our humidifier and Tempur-Pedic mattress.

I ask him, "If you can't adapt to a new environment for ten days, how are you going to live here permanently?"

My reactive anger is deep-seated because this scenario represents our largest struggle when it comes to taking leaps: my insistence and Jamie's resistance. It resurfaces my year of IVF hell and the morning that Jamie complained about bringing his sperm sample to the hospital. But unlike IVF, moving is something that we can work equally toward, and I need to know that Jamie will do his part.

"Are you having second thoughts about moving?" I ask.

"No," Jamie says. "I just wish you'd be more sympathetic that it's going to be really different for me. It's not going to be easy."

And I think, *Has anything we've ever sought been easy?*

Chapter

44

Because we've decided to move to Chicago, naturally, we come home to a leaking roof and water stains on our ceilings.

I'm surprised I didn't see it coming. Did I really think that, unlike trying to have a baby, this would be a smooth process? It's like fate is shaking its finger and saying, "Not so fast."

When we bought our house, the one visible side of our roof looked relatively new. We thought we wouldn't have to worry about new shingles for at least another ten years. But then, after we moved in, Jamie was painting our bedroom, and he felt dampness on the wall. Then the pipe-seal around our cast-iron stove bubbled up. Then a water spot sprouted on our guest bedroom ceiling.

Jamie's contractor friend climbed up onto the roof and discovered that the other half of the peak was a good thirty years old—the shingles blown off, the tar exposed. It turns out that the previous owners had only installed half of a new roof on the side that's visible from the street, and our inspector had never climbed a ladder to investigate it.

Jamie's friend did his best to tar the bald spots, getting us through the rainy season. The following winter was a mild one, and we had our ceilings patched and repainted to hide the sagging seams. We got roof quotes, but then I got pregnant, and we had Geo and we never came up with that extra $7,000 we needed for a new roof.

So, when we come home from Chicago to find water damage, it's not just here and there, but striping and spotting our ceiling like a mixture of zebra and leopard print.

Somehow, we need to come up with the money. There's no ignoring the issue anymore. So now, in addition to finding new jobs in Chicago and landing a spacious, affordable apartment, we have to lay down a fresh roof before we can even think about putting our house on the market.

Since I can't pull seven thousand dollars out of my ass, I concentrate on things I have a bit more control over—jobs and apartments. I email my friends for help. They reply immediately with recruiters' names and apartment listings. The pictures of modern two-bedrooms excite me, and I can't help but fantasize about our new life in Chicago.

I know that I am seriously pursuing this, but what about Jamie? Like any other decision I've ever made, I want it to happen now, and I am putting all of my energy into lining up the details. But Jamie moves slowly, methodically. He usually takes months just to pick out electronics and kitchen gadgets. He has to think out every step of the process and troubleshoot possible obstacles.

It occurs to me that even though we agreed to move, we never agreed on a timeline. I would be happy to wake up in Chicago tomorrow, but Jamie might be thinking of this as a two-year goal. And I've learned from past experience that the more pressure I put on a situation, the more Jamie hesitates. He wants things to be stress-free, even if it will take longer.

How best to ease into the conversation? I wonder as I sauté sausage and peppers for dinner.

When I walk into our bedroom to announce that supper is ready, Jamie is changing out of work clothes and Geo's propped on our bed, batting at Tessa. *What have I got to lose?* I think. I climb onto the bed and pull Geo onto my lap, then ready myself.

"So I've been looking at apartments . . ." I say to Jamie's back as he bends over to take off his socks. "And I think we can actually get some of the things that we don't have here—like two bathrooms and a new kitchen . . ."

"Yeah," Jamie says. "That's assuming I find a job making the same salary I do now." He throws his socks into the hamper.

I take a deep breath for patience against the sarcasm that coats all of his words.

"Well, Courtney gave me the info for two headhunters and I don't know if you want to go down this route, but Theresa sent me the name of a guy who might be able to get you a chef job at his restaurant."

"Oh yeah? A chef? Making, what? Sixteen bucks an hour?" Jamie says.

And so comes the explosion.

It gets the best of us—his over-practicality versus my unrealistic dreaming, his cynicism versus my defensiveness.

Me: Why can't you see the positive in anything?

Him: I'm just talking things out. This is the reality.

Me: You can't adapt. You're terrified of risk.

Him: Why? Because I have genuine concerns?

Me: No, because you talk yourself out of life.

Him: This is who I am. You know this. I'm logical, Nadine.

All the while, from my lap, Geo watches everything. This is the scene I promised myself would never happen—for Jamie and I to fight in front of our precious boy. But like so many other things I've sworn against, here the moment is, playing out on the stage of our bedroom. Geo wriggles his torso and flaps his arms, but he doesn't cry. Maybe he thinks we are playing a game, like the way we bark at Tess to make her bark back. Or maybe he does need to see this, to know that disagreements are inevitable.

Jamie sighs, annoyed.

"OK, Nadine," he says with mocking surrender. "What do you want me to do? Just 'yes' you? Then that's what I'll do. I'll 'yes' you to death. Apparently you've thought everything through. So, whatever you want to do, we'll do. Is that what you want?"

"No," I say, but I think, *Maybe it is. Maybe I do want to hear Yes. Maybe I want to hear Yes, I'll move for you, and Yes, I'll do it without complaint, and Yes, I'll even do it with excitement, because, Nadine, that's what you did for me.*

Two days later, I'm doing my usual morning straightening up in the living room when I trip over the trap-shooting equipment Jamie got for Christmas. Geo crawls after me and Tess after Geo as I walk into the kitchen to ask Jamie where he'd like me to move the box.

"It doesn't matter. I probably have to return it," he says, hurriedly, while packing his lunch. "Where am I going to use it in Chicago?"

And, just like that, our feud resumes—his negativity, my fantasies. I point out that he's only been shooting a handful of times in the past two years because his friends never commit, and that maybe, in Chicago, he'll have my friends' husbands to go with. Then he asks if he can store his drums at my parents' because there will be no place for them in an apartment—a valid question, but I'm too pissed off at this point to respond civilly.

He can't say, "I'm sad that I have to make sacrifices," and I can't say, "I understand your sadness."

Because that's what it all boils down to, doesn't it—sacrifice and sadness? In a marriage, in parenthood, how much do we sacrifice for another person's happiness before it leads to our own sadness? It feels like our last three years have been some kind of grueling experiment in this very issue. I'm actually surprised it has taken this long for the stress of it all to catch up with us.

When Jamie closes the door to leave for work, I'm left in the silence. Geo crawls over to Tessa's water dish and dumps it over onto himself. My immediate instinct is to yell out, "God damn it," and, right then, I see how very, very easy it is to become the stressed-out, screaming parent.

So, instead, I put all of my angry energy into smothering Geo with kisses, as if these smooches might protect him from my unhappiness. I consider reconciling with Jamie, but when I look out at the driveway, his spot is empty, and only the exhaust fumes linger.

Over the next couple of weeks, our arguments continue. Though they are decreasingly explosive, they still sting.

I say that we'll have to sell one of our cars when we move in order to save money, and Jamie says, "You're not single anymore. You're really going to take a baby on an L-train?"

Next he asks, "How are we going to live in a loud apartment when Geo goes to bed at eight every night?"

I see what he's getting at. We have an ideal life in Whitinsville—a three-bedroom house with a huge fenced-in yard, a pool, two cars, woods for roaming, strip malls for shopping. Who wouldn't want that? Why would I want to make life harder? Why would I want to downsize to one car and a two-bedroom apartment with noisy neighbors and no yard? When everybody else usually does city life when they're single and the burbs when they have a family, why do I want to do the opposite?

Because, I reason, *this life, as ideal as it seems, is so very, very isolated that I know that no matter how many logical reasons Jamie gives me, my heart will still feel the same.*

Because, on Friday night, on my way home from yoga, when I drive through our little town, past the neighbor's junkyard and the boarded-up mill buildings, I declare to the air, "I will not miss you, or you, or you," and I fantasize about having art galleries and coffee shops within walking distance.

Because, when the wide-open weekend stretches ahead, its only highlight a trip to the strip mall, I imagine what it will be like to have my sister and girlfriends within a five-mile radius—to eat Sunday dinner together, to celebrate birthdays together. Together.

Because, if I let myself sit and think, I get the scary feeling that there is a life somewhere else waiting for me, and the longer I stay in this small town, the further away that life drifts. And even now that we've made the decision to move, it still feels like that other life has floated so far away that it might be impossible to catch it.

Chapter

45

Yesterday, we stopped for gas, and Jamie got out to pump. I watched him walk around to Geo's window, on the opposite side of the gas tank, just to beam at him. Jamie's eyes crinkled and he smiled his crooked smile—the one he used to use on me that means he's so happy that he could tear up. Through the window, he mouthed *I love you* to our sweet boy and it made me want to tear up too, but for different reasons.

"You look at him so lovingly," I said when Jamie got back in the car. I hid my jealousy and the words, "the way you used to look at me."

We said that we'd never be like them—the unaffectionate, bickering couple.

No. Not us. Never. Yet . . . isn't that what we've become?

And the saddest part of all? *We're* responsible for the sour state of our relationship. It happened because we wanted it all. We wanted to live together, but with cohabitation came resentment that one of us had to leave our life behind. We wanted the wedding, but alongside it came the stress of pleasing everyone and getting a loan to cover the costs. We wanted a house, but by signing the purchase and sale agreement we also agreed to endless repairs and a mortgage. We wanted a baby, but that meant IVF horrors and failed pregnancy attempts. And now, we want happiness, but that entails moving across the country and starting a new life. We keep wanting more, *More*, MORE, and in the process, we've lost ourselves.

Why has every seemingly good decision brought equal measures of hardship?

In the montage we envision of the next stage of life, we only see the blissful moments—how living together means sleeping with limbs entwined, how a wedding means a white dress and a slow dance, how a house means planting a garden, how a baby means snuggling up and reading books.

But here I am with it all—the ring on my finger, the roof over my head, the baby in my arms, and I'm slamming the basement door because Jamie has forgotten for the twentieth time to close it behind him, and if Geo crawls on the floor, he'll tumble to his death. And here Jamie is, grumbling as he searches for pacifiers that I never put back in the same spot.

At night, we're un-showered and exhausted and short on patience and so entirely spent from washing bottles and changing diapers and preparing to put our house on the market that we have no energy for ourselves, let alone each other. We collapse into bed and we retreat. Almost simultaneously, we place items into our ears to tune out—ear plugs for me, ear buds for him. I search for reprieve in books, he in DVDs. Both of us make sporadic attempts at being affectionate. But after two minutes of rubbing each other's arms, we fall asleep. Like a diet with too little calories coming in, it's completely unsustainable to exert ourselves any further. We're completely depleted and defeated.

I've spent so much of my life wanting to speed ahead, but now I want to slow down. Way down. Some days I want to reverse.

I'm so incredibly sad for this thing that we can't seem to get back. I drive to work and well up thinking of this precious vanished gift. *I want it back,* I demand to someone, no one. I want my fresh face and alert eyes, but even if I could barter for time reversal, more than my youth, there's one thing that I want above all else: I want to be the woman that Jamie fell in love with. I want for him to look at me the way he used to. I want for him to touch the small of my back when we're standing in line. I want us to hold hands for entire car rides. I want to catch him in my periphery, gazing at me like there's no one more amazing on the planet. I want him to look at me through the car window and mouth *I love you.*

I have to do something. The state of our marriage depends on it. After all, Jamie used to send me cards because I sent them to him. He touched my back because I rubbed his scalp. He held my hand because I reached for it. And when was the last time I did any of these things? In fact, two mornings in a row now, I've smothered Geo with kisses, then walked right past Jamie, forgetting to say goodbye.

And Jamie looked at me with such pained neglect that I know I'm not the only one feeling this loss.

If I want Jamie to be more complimentary to me, I realize, I must be more complimentary to him. So, I send him a text that says, *You're a great dad. I love you.*

And, to my surprise, he types back instantly:
Thank you sweety, I love you too.

The universe tilts the scales in our favor. We secure a bank loan, and the January air warms to a balmy forty-five degrees for two days.

The roofers—a ragtag crew—pound and scrape until the old shingles litter the melting snow on our front lawn. The noise and debris drive Geo and me from the house, but it's OK, because we come back home to magnificent leakproof shingles.

For Jamie and me, it feels like we've also undergone some repairs. The day the roof is completed, our shoulders release and we exhale deeply. Finally, we have one less thing to worry about.

That night, after we put Geo to bed, we go about our evening routines. Jamie loads the dishwasher, and I wash my face. When Jamie sinks into his chair and clicks on the TV, I sit on his lap and kiss him, parting my mouth. He opens his, and I slide my tongue across his teeth, then suck his bottom lip. His hands cup my face, and I kiss him harder, working my fingers through his hair. And because it's been so very long—weeks, maybe a month—since we've made love or even kissed like this, it feels new.

So, I make this my vow—*Pretend like it's new. Pretend like you're seducing him for the first time, and you have no worries, no responsibilities, no bills to pay, no house to sell, no emotional baggage weighing you down.*

We kiss like we're exploring each other. My body buzzes, and I feel his responding, too.

"What's that?" I joke as I rub my hand across his lap.

I get up and say that I'm going upstairs if he'd like to join me.

The electric candle in our bedroom window spreads a soft glow across the bed as we undress and crawl under our warm blankets. The sound machine emits waves of oceanic white noise. Even Tessa must feel the romance brewing, because she retreats to the guest bedroom, giving us our privacy.

Jamie kisses my neck, giving me goose bumps, and works his mouth down to my chest. He wasn't able to caress it when I was nursing, so this sensation also feels like new. He presses his lips to my skin until every centimeter of my body tingles.

Then he slides his fingers over my belly button and between my legs.

When he rubs me, I tremble, and when his fingers enter me, he swirls them, grazing the loveliest of spots.

We kiss hard, our tongues tickling the roofs of each other's mouths. I nibble on his neck and moan, gripping his back until my nails dig in. My body convulses, and I slide on top of him.

I arch my back and rock my hips while he grips my waist. We whisper to each other words of raw desire. The wanting is so deep between us that Jamie moves in ways he's never moved before, and I say things I've never said before. We feel young again.

We go round after round until we are panting and sore in the best of ways.

Afterward, we splay out and catch our breaths. Then Jamie slides me over to him, curling his body around mine.

We fall asleep, naked and content.

Chapter

46

Our realtor, Christine, sits at our dining room table and flips through a bound packet of house listings. A box of photographs occupies the space next to her—evidence of our meager efforts to pack up things we won't need for the next few months.

"Here's your house, as it was advertised when you bought it," she says, pointing to the listing of the *Little Women* house that caught my eye on a cold March afternoon four years ago.

Jamie and I marvel at the pictures of the maroon walls and the stained beige carpet, now long gone. We've fenced in the yard, stripped the wallpaper, painted the rooms, pulled up the carpet, put down new floors, replaced the furnace, installed new plumbing, remodeled the bathroom, and laid a new roof, which is why we both reason that the house should be worth at least $230,000. We owe $202,000 on it, and after closing costs, *and* the realtors' commissions, *and* paying back the roof loan, we need a little left over to cover our moving costs. Our savings account is nonexistent, so if we are offered anything lower, we won't be able to sell.

Christine flips to the next page, which displays the handful of houses for sale in our town. All of them have been on the market for at least three months. All of them have had to drop their asking prices. I swallow and glance at Jamie. He bounces Geo on his knee to hide his anxiety.

The next page shows an updated three-bedroom that's comparable to ours, but it also boasts two things ours doesn't—a remodeled kitchen and a garage.

"So, you can see here that they listed this house for $229 and it sold for $218. Which is why I think that you'd get between $220 and $210 for this house."

"But we bought it at $209," I argue.

"Unfortunately," Christine says, "what the bank will give the buyers is based on what the other houses in the area are selling for."

Our improvements and the rising market—none of this matters—she explains, because Worcester County is still suffering from short sales and foreclosures.

After she leaves, I put Geo in his high chair and break up bits of puffs. Jamie cuts up kielbasa in the kitchen, then walks into the dining room to find me staring at the table, my jaw set. My entire body is stone. Geo slaps his tray for more puffs with increasing intensity, and I must steady my breathing as I shake out the cereal.

"Nader," Jamie says as he crouches down beside my chair. "Look at me."

I look over his shoulder at the window that leads to this godforsaken town that is crushing my dreams. Jamie sweeps my hair out of my eyes and says, "We will make it to Chicago. We've got a good thing going here." He gestures at himself and me and Geo, who hoots as if on cue. We both laugh, and I wipe my eyes.

"We can't let the stress of this get the best of us," Jamie says and he kisses me so gently that I know that we're in this together. I'm reminded of the feeling we shared early on in our relationship—the feeling that when two people are in love, they can conquer the world. *And,* I ask myself, *in the past eight years together, hasn't this power resurfaced again and again when we needed it most? Haven't we faced obstacle after obstacle, only to overcome each? The long distance, the IVF, the hydronephrosis, the raising of Geo alone—hasn't this all just been conditioning us to surmount our biggest obstacle yet?*

So, I repeat this to myself now as a mantra. *We can conquer the world . . . We can conquer the world . . .* Or at the very least, *We can conquer Whitinsville.*

Chapter

47

The winter is relentless, record breaking. It's still snowing heavily in March as we prep the house to go on the market. As Jamie nails trim and installs a banister, I think of him, last year, assembling Geo's crib, laying down new carpet in the nursery. I reminisce, but sometimes the reminiscing makes Jamie sad. Though he is getting the house ready and is happy that we'll have help with Geo in Chicago, it doesn't mean the transition isn't hard for him. He looks at Geo's cozy room and our huge yard and goes quiet. He talks about getting Geo a swing set, as if he has forgotten that we won't be living here when Geo is old enough to enjoy it.

What I can't admit is that, like him, when I rock Geo to sleep in the glider at night and stare out his skylight at the moon, I am similarly sad for all we will leave behind. Like Jamie, I shudder just thinking of another family setting down their furniture where ours used to be, replacing our memories with their own.

Even purging and packing pains me more than I expect. The realtor tells us to "thin out" our space—a.k.a. declutter and depersonalize—so I have taken down almost every sentimental item: the colorfully embroidered table runner from Guatemala, the collage of Jamie and me from our first year of dating looking young and slim and tan and huddled close, so very in love. Side tables and chests have been stored in the basement, vases given to Goodwill. My beloved books go into boxes.

When I stow away our wedding album and pictures, Jamie goes into the basement and brings our portrait back upstairs and stands it up on the Winthrop desk in our dining room. I bring our wedding album back up and set that out as well. Depersonalizing the house feels like deleting our past. And taking down pictures of Geo feels even worse. He's not even a year old, and we're already erasing evidence of his existence. I have a picture of him doing yoga from our baby-mama class. He's wearing a yellow sweater-vest and doing locust pose. I think about that period of time—before we were burdened by the stress of selling our house, when I got to spend my Wednesday mornings in a yoga studio, sitting v-legged with other women, our babies looking up at us from the mats.

I didn't know how precious those moments were.

Instead of storing the photo away with the many others in our basement, I move it to the side of the fridge. If the realtor tells me to "thin it out," I'm going to thin her out.

On a Saturday in early April, the three of us get into the car and drive to the zoo. We don't pack or clean or job search or work on the yard. We leave it all behind for a day of ease. The ground is thawing, and the field that acts as the zoo parking lot is muddy. But the air is warm enough that we can leave our jackets in the car. We feel light as we push Geo's stroller through the entrance. Despite the dull ground and cloudy sky, we are struck by color. Tulips have started to sprout along the fence. A large macaw perches on a branch while a peacock fans its tail. Geo points at everything, and Jamie takes him out of his stroller to get a better view. I stand back and take a picture of them: Jamie carrying Geo on his shoulders, Geo wrapping his arms around Jamie's forehead. Their love is brighter than any feather or flower here.

Lately, I've been mourning everything I lost when I moved to Massachusetts, but life's gift is here before me in all of its abundant glory.

Geo is so remarkable that I stare at him most days, baffled by his existence. Jamie and I look at him during dinner as he sits in his high chair shoving pieces of rice into his mouth, and we shake our heads.

"We created that," Jamie says.

And I say, "I don't believe it."

Because I don't. I can't imagine that I ever did enough good in this world to deserve the life before us.

There's not much beyond Geo's eye shape and dimples that connects his appearance to mine, but I'll be damned if we don't have similar personalities. Geo wails to be fed and I can't whip up food fast enough. He eyes a teething ring and grumbles like a gremlin if I don't hand it to him with urgency.

"I wonder where he gets his impatience from," Jamie jokes sometimes.

I laugh and say, "He got some good traits from me too, ya know."

In grocery stores and restaurants, Geo follows patrons with his eyes, and I can see that he has my knack for observing others.

But I'm most proud when Geo pulls himself up onto the couch and shimmies along it, grunting and attempting to walk. Jamie will say, "He's determined like his mama." And I feel my chest expand, because maybe that's what got us this baby. Even if I am not the most patient person in the world, I sure as hell tried everything I could.

And, maybe, the universe decided, that was enough.

Now, at the zoo, I snap a picture and join them, rubbing Jamie's back, then Geo's.

"What do you think about having his first birthday here?" I ask Jamie as we near the wooden party pavilions.

Geo points at the picnic tables, communicating that he wants to get closer. He sees the birthday banners and points some more. We laugh and ask him if this would be a fun place for his birthday. He reaches up to touch the banner, then claps.

"Well, I think that settles it," Jamie says.

Chapter

48

"Will we need these anytime soon?" Jamie and I ask each other about the clothes and toys Geo has outgrown. I think about being pregnant again while trying to settle into Chicago, and I shake my head. Jamie talks about how hard it would be to give our attention to two children right now. So we sell the stuff, deciding, silently, that we're not going to have a second child in the near future. We sell Geo's swing to a consignment store, staring sadly as the worker shoves it into the heap of rockers and bassinets. The forty-six dollars doesn't seem like nearly enough for the memories of Geo swaying peacefully during his naps.

And what about the remaining embryos we have in storage? What should we do with them?

Each time we get the bill from the cryo lab, Jamie asks me what I'd like to do. He's ready to cancel, but I've been resistant because it feels scary not to have a backup plan in case we want more kids later. But then, something shifts in me, and I tell Jamie that I'm ready, too.

Because we lost two embryos to the thaw before the transfer, and the two that were transferred didn't survive, there are five left. Jamie and I have discussed, ad nauseam, all of the reasons for canceling storage: *It's expensive. They are grade-C embryos; they'd likely not survive anyway. As of now, we only want one child. If we wanted a second, it wouldn't be for at least another couple of years, and by then, the embryos would be five years old—what some doctors consider their expiration date.*

I think of a friend, who, after having a healthy son, had two miscarriages. And I think about how the miscarriage must feel for someone like her as opposed to someone who has never had kids. When she loses a child in the first trimester, she is not losing a twelve-week-old fetus. She has merely to look at her healthy son and see that a fetus grows into an infant, who grows into a toddler, who grows into a teenager, who grows into a man.

It's not until we sign the embryo discard consent forms that I look at Geo and realize that we've just discarded five possible adult lives.

That night and the next, every time I look at Geo, I see the faces of Raya, and Lucy, and Ty, and Percy, and Ariana. But I don't call to reverse our decision, and by the time I do pick up the phone, my fingers refuse to press "call."

I think of Mom thirty years ago, pregnant with me and ready to dial the abortion clinic, then hanging up.

And here I am, agreeing to the opposite decision.

Here's why: because, though I am mourning our children, I don't yearn to see their toys sprawled across our floors, and I don't listen for their voices calling out to me.

With Geo on my hip, I walk toward our living room, dodging his toy trucks and trains. When I put him down, he stands against the couch. He reaches his hand out to me.

"Mama," he says.

And the sentence comes to my brain, clear in a way that is so rare.

I don't want anything else, it says.

It's enough. It's more than enough. It's so much that I feel undeserving. And I want to enjoy it. I want, for once, to take it easy. In Chicago, I want to have *less*: *less* house, *less* yard, *less* responsibility and only *more* of the important things—friends, family, love.

Is this how long it has taken me, I think, *to stop chasing it, whatever "it" is? To feel full? To realize that I need to pause and be grateful for what I have?*

How hard I forced life to beat the message into my stubborn brain.

But, I think, *what if, next year, we change our minds and we want another child but we don't have the same luck that we had with Geo? What if, by choosing to stop the storage, we've just chosen to deny ourselves any more children?*

Another clear sentence resonates.

I can't go through it all again.

Though I've always tried to prove myself and my strength, I surrender to this. It's bigger than me, and it's more than I can handle. How often I've said "yes" to everything and gotten in over my head. How often the sacrifice of saying "yes" has hurt me. And this decision hurts me too, but, finally, I'm saying "no."

I'm cleaning out my dresser when I discover my moratorium of IVF memories: the no-skid hospital socks, my good-luck necklace, the extra syringes and medication, our embryo picture.

Geo crawls around my feet. He stands, holding the nightstand knob, and bangs happily on the wood. He knows nothing of the journey. I could just throw all of this stuff away and try to forget that it all happened. Often enough, it feels like it was some other woman who pricked herself with needles and took pills and marked calendars and cried at every menstrual cycle and almost bled to death. If I throw these things out, maybe I could do the same to the bad memories, as well.

Instead, I sit down on the floor next to Geo and pull him into my lap.

And I begin to describe each item.

In fact, I'm telling our story a lot these days. It's unavoidable. When I compose a writing advice column or talk about Geo with his pediatrician, the story is innately woven into our history. I'm speaking at a conference on a panel about mothers who write, and my experiences of trying to become a mother are so much a part of my being that I feel I must talk about it.

What baffles me is that the more I talk about infertility with people, the more they talk about it with me. After the conference, three different women come up to me to share their IVF stories.

When I share my experience with some mothers in my moms' group, a handful of them confess that they have also gone to fertility clinics.

A colleague's daughter, a woman at the grocery store, a fellow writer, a neighbor—they've all been through some form of reproductive assistance.

Two of my Chicago friends go through IVF—one gets pregnant and the other does not, but even my "lucky" friend who conceives gets a blood clot and hyperstimulation that lands her in the hospital. She has to take blood thinners and have liters of fluid drained from her abdomen. When our other friends say they can't believe what the conception-journey can do to a person, I say, "I can."

All along, I thought I was alone. I thought I was one of the rare women for whom IVF was unsuccessful, and even rarer for the near-fatal complications I experienced. But what I'm realizing now is that I am not alone. Men and women everywhere struggle with infertility and have equally painful stories to share. But they have hopeful stories too.

Being on the other side doesn't actually make me feel victorious or wise. In fact, most of the time, I feel guilty for miraculously having a baby when these child-seeking women are no less deserving than I.

But I do feel something else: camaraderie. Despite our various backgrounds, we all share something.

And so, as they speak of the testing and the disappointments, I nod and pat their arms. I hug them—friends and strangers—because we are all soldiers in the same war.

Chapter

49

Along with forsythia, good fortune sprouts at our doorstep. I get a remote job as a curriculum writer, and Jamie applies to a company in Chicago who like him so much they offer to hold the position until August, so that, hopefully, our house will sell in the meantime.

We've talked together about the type of apartment we want—a two-bedroom in a central location with a parking spot and an in-unit washer-dryer. Jamie would love a newer kitchen, and we'd both like to live in a low-rise that seems more like a town house. I've Googled "family-friendly neighborhoods in Chicago" and made a list of the top five.

There's one catch, though. When I go on Zillow to see what's out there, there's nothing in our price range that meets all of our desires. There are some nice places, but either they're not dog friendly, or they're in a high-rise, or they're so far away from the center of things that it'd be like living in Whitinsville all over again.

Jamie's future company asks that he fly to Chicago so that they can meet him in person, and Geo and I join him so that we can also use the time to search for apartments. On Friday night in our Chicago hotel, I'm desperately searching online to find apartments we can look at the next day, and I see that one of the contacts at the bottom of an ad is my friend Kristin from high school. I email her at 1:00 a.m. and, shockingly, she messages right back. She tells us about new construction in Ravenswood, which is a neighborhood on my "family-friendly neighborhoods" list.

Ravenswood is on the north side of the city, near parks and beaches and restaurants and baby play-centers, away from the chaos of the Loop and bar scene of Wrigleyville. The apartments are dog friendly with an in-unit washer-dryer and a modern kitchen. They're going fast, but Kristin calls in a favor and we get an appointment for the next day at noon.

As Mom watches Geo back at our hotel, Jamie and I pull up to the new complex and smile. The low-rise apartments are made to look like town houses. They have little gardens everywhere and a long courtyard where Geo can run around safely. Right down the street is a brand-new grocery store. Now we just hope that the inside will look as nice as the outside.

The leasing manager opens the door to the model unit and Jamie and I walk in slowly, marveling at the place. The living room has tons of windows and an open floor plan to the kitchen and dining room. Geo would be able to play in sight as we prepare dinner. Jamie runs his hand along the island in the center of the kitchen and says, "This would be a nice space to make dinner."

The master bedroom has walls of shelving, two large closets, and its own bathroom. The second bedroom is large, with enough room for Geo's crib and a bed so that Massachusetts friends can visit or Mom can sleep over when she babysits. A cozy balcony looks out toward the center courtyard.

There is nothing *Little Women*-esque about it. As much as I loved the idea of the March family residence, I realize that I had it in Whitinsville, and the weight of its upkeep, of its country isolation, caused me more sadness than joy. Here, the walls are white; the tiles are new. There's no history, no expectation. It's a completely clean slate, no idealistic version of "home" to live up to. Best of all, there are no old roofs to replace. If something breaks, it's no longer our responsibility. It's evident, now, that when I watched *Little Women* as a little girl, what I pined after wasn't actually a New England colonial home, but the feeling it evoked—warmth and love, togetherness—things that are up to me to create. And the story line I had loved so much of a woman pursuing her dreams was something I'd neglected during my quest. Now, it all seems possible again: to reclaim my city, to write my heart out.

Jamie and I don't even have to ask each other if we want the place. Right away, we start discussing which unit to choose and where our furniture will go. More and more people arrive, looking at different units, and we know we have to act fast if we want to secure an apartment. We run to the bank to get half a month's rent, then come back to fill out the paperwork.

Afterward, we drive around exploring the neighborhood and holding hands over the center console. There's a day-care center down the road and a park with a walking trail just two blocks away. At the corner, there's a restaurant called—fittingly enough—Gio's.

This neighborhood and this apartment are the opposite of everything I've known for the last six years, of what Jamie has known for the last forty. And, though I'm ecstatic about it, and Jamie seems to be as well, I know from being on the other end that things won't always go this smoothly. Everything won't always fall into place. I know that, one day, Jamie might look out at the horizon and wish to see mountains or an ocean. I know that, on Friday nights, he may yearn to hang out with his friends. I know that he might hear L trains and taxis and long for the silence of the suburbs. I know that, in Chicago, he may never truly feel at home. And I too might rock Geo in his new room and miss looking at the moon through the skylight. I'm sure that when I sip wine with my Chicago friends, I'll wish that Kelly and Kate and Jenn were among them.

That night, as we have drinks at Courtney's apartment, I get to catch up with Marie and see Theresa's baby bump. I'm smiling so hard that my cheeks hurt, but what about Jamie? Now that we've put money on a new place and have an August move-in date, things are really happening. But in the mad dash to secure the apartment and get to Courtney's, we haven't had much time to talk about how he's handling it all.

But when I look over at him, he's sitting at Courtney's dining room table, proudly showing the video of the model unit to my friends.

The next morning, Jamie and I show my sister and her boyfriend our new building, then we walk around Lincoln Square—a nearby area that's lined with coffee shops and specialty stores. All around us, couples walk dogs and push strollers, enjoying the warm weather. As we wander down the street, I kiss Geo, who's strapped to me in a carrier, and I tell him about our future neighborhood. He smiles, pointing at things and asking, "That? That?" I explain what each thing is: a restaurant, a fountain, a music school, a playground. Geo stares, inquisitively, processing it all. He no longer thinks like a baby, nor does he look like one either. With his wispy blonde hair and prominent nose, his features have become more pronounced, as has his personality. He babbles and claps, and I realize that when we move here in a couple months, he'll have achieved other milestones, too. He'll be a walking, talking toddler.

Jamie points out different restaurants he'd like to go to. "That looks good," he says, excitedly, then we walk into a shop that offers cooking class, and Jamie lights up about being able to teach there.

I can sense that his enthusiasm is genuine. As I look at his face and Geo's—almost an exact replica—I see the same enthusiasm. Though we know, all too well, that nothing is a guarantee, that everything can end in "for now," in this moment, we are happy, and I hope that they will like our new city when we move here as much as they seem to like it now.

I envision our very near future—walking along this street and taking Geo to a music class after breakfast or taking Tessa to the dog-friendly beach nearby. I envision Mom and Dana watching Geo so that I can write at a coffee shop or Jamie and I can go on a date, hold hands, maybe even steal a kiss. And I feel finally at peace. We have made the right decision for our family.

Of this much I'm sure.

Chapter

50

Ours is by far the most vibrant out of all the birthday party pavilions at the zoo. Blow-up giraffes and zebras hang from the rafters. Our guests moo and oink as they don animal masks.

We all take turns riding the merry-go-round—Kelly and Daphne, Ciara and Lily, Jenn and Mateo, me and Geo. Jamie's parents help serve food. Mom snaps pictures, and Dana joins us via FaceTime.

The May sun peeks out and sprinkles confetti on us, warming our smiling cheeks.

After eating sandwiches and blowing bubbles, we can't put it off any longer. It's time to sing happy birthday to our little boy.

Behind us is the banner Jamie made at work containing a picture for every month of Geo's life. Before us, sitting at picnic tables, are all the people who have accompanied us on this long, long journey.

Our healthy, grinning, birthday-hatted boy sits in his high chair with a cupcake on his tray. Atop the white frosting is a big blue G. There is no candle, because somehow in the chaos of decorating the pavilion, I lost it. I've searched the garbage bags and crumpled wrapping paper, but I can't find the wax number-one anywhere.

Jamie and I stand together, looking at our son, and when we begin to sing, we both get choked up. Memories of the past year fizz to the surface of my mind: Geo swaddled and wearing his yellow knit hat at the hospital, him rolling over for the first time, him kissing us with his big open mouth, him grunting and rocking and finally crawling, him feeding himself and clapping, him kicking his legs happily when we walk into a room.

Jamie blinks back tears, too, and I wonder if he's remembering the same moments. We finish our last "Happy Birthday to you . . ." but there's no candle to blow. And in that instant, I'm glad for it.

There's no wishing for anything.

No hoping that the couple who is coming to visit our house tomorrow will buy it, or that our apartment in the city will be the scene of many good moments to come, or that our marriage will stay strong, or that we will be able to give Geo a sibling later on if we decide to.

There's just this moment: Geo, in his birthday hat and birthday bib, swiping the icing with his hand, then smashing the cake, and in the most generous of gestures, reaching over and offering us the feast on his sticky fingers.

We eat the bits of cake from his hand, then, covered in blue icing, Jamie and I kiss each other. Jamie pulls back and smiles at me—his crooked smile, just for me. We kneel next to Geo and Mom snaps a picture: the image I foresaw when I was twenty-two and giddy in love, when I was twenty-seven and buying the Vitello bib in Italy, when I was twenty-nine and contracting in a sunny hospital room in Newton: Me and Jamie, and sitting between us, our blonde-haired, blue-eyed boy.

Acknowledgments

I am eternally grateful to my love, Jamie Johnstone, who cooked our meals and watched our son during my many long writing days. You bravely gave your blessing for me to write about our intimate moments in these pages. Thank you for always believing in me and in us.

Geo Johnstone, my Boo Bear, I love you through and through.

Mom, you have and would do anything for us, and your generosity never goes unnoticed. One of the many great gifts you passed on to me was the motivation to remain driven, even in the face of adversity, which is why this book exists today.

Dana, you are the best listener I know. Thank you for always hearing me out and never judging me. You are an amazing woman and my best friend.

To the Johnstones (Mumsie, Poppy, Josh, Ciara, and Lily) thank you for your love and understanding during that challenging and emotional period of our lives.

The Kenneys: While I was on the East Coast, I felt your love every time I made Irish bread.

The title and main message of this book came from our doula, Amy. You brought our hope and our son to life.

To my friends in Boston and Chicago: Stef Coleman, Jenn De Leon, Jenny Dierolf, Cheryl Gilchrist, Amy Jakubiak, Kelly Lazlo, Stephanie Leopold, Katy Lupo, Sarah Neubauer, Theresa O'Brien, Kelly Steel, Kate Wisel, and Courtney Wonneberg. You are such powerful, hilarious, honest women and you push me to be my best self.

Jeanine, our sessions got me through the pain so that I could write about it.

My talented teachers at Columbia College Chicago made

me a writer. Special thanks to Patty McNair, Joe Meno, Alexis Pride, and Megan Stielstra. You kicked my butt.

To Grub Street in Boston and Story Studio in Chicago. You have been the literary support groups that have fostered my writing career.

To agent extraordinaire, Emma Patterson: you had faith in this book from the start. Thank you for your encouragement and keen editorial eye.

She Writes Press, you made my book dreams come true.

I wrote most of this book at the Montrose and Wolcott Starbucks in Ravenswood while listening to Eric Church and Fleetwood Mac. Thank you, Madison and crew, for letting me stay all day and refilling my water bottle a million times. Your smiling faces and mocha syrup got me through the hardest of writing days.

Cheryl Strayed and Mary Karr, my favorite memoirists—I reread *Wild* and *Lit* a dozen times throughout the writing of this book to remind myself how the masters do it.

Last but not least, to everyone fighting the infertility battle, I will pass on to you the same words that were passed onto us:

You will have your baby. Of this much I'm sure.

About the Author

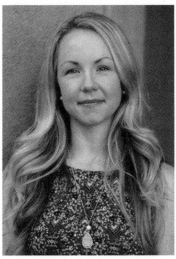

photo credit: Chris Loomis

NADINE KENNEY JOHNSTONE teaches writing at Loyola University and received her MFA from Columbia College Chicago. Her work has been featured in *Chicago* magazine, *The Moth, PANK,* and various anthologies, including *The Magic of Memoir.* Nadine is a writing coach who presents at conferences internationally. She lives near Chicago with her family.

www.nadinekenneyjohnstone.com

SELECTED TITLES FROM SHE WRITES PRESS

She Writes Press is an independent publishing company
founded to serve women writers everywhere.
Visit us at www.shewritespress.com.

The Doctor and The Stork: A Memoir of Modern Medical Babymaking by
K.K. Goldberg. $16.95, 978-1-63152-830-9. A mother's compelling
story of her post-IVF, high-risk pregnancy with twins—the very
definition of a modern medical babymaking experience.

Make a Wish for Me: A Mother's Memoir by LeeAndra Chergey. $16.95,
978-1-63152-828-6. A life-changing diagnosis teaches a family that
where's there is love there is hope—and that being "normal" is not
nearly as important as providing your child with a life full of joy,
love, and acceptance.

Breathe: A Memoir of Motherhood, Grief, and Family Conflict by Kelly
Kittel. $16.95, 978-1-938314-78-0. A mother's heartbreaking account
of losing two sons in the span of nine months—and learning, despite
all the obstacles in her way, to find joy in life again.

Splitting the Difference: A Heart-Shaped Memoir by Tré Miller-
Rodríguez. $19.95, 978-1-938314-20-9. When 34-year-old Tré
Miller-Rodríguez's husband dies suddenly from a heart attack, her
grief sends her on an unexpected journey that culminates in a reun-
ion with the biological daughter she gave up at 18.

Changed By Chance: My Journey of Triumph Over Tragedy by Elizabeth
Barker. $16.95, 978-1-63152-810-1. When her dreams of parenthood
and becoming a career mom take a nightmarish twist, Elizabeth
Barker has to learn how to summon her inner warrior—for her and
her family's survival.

Three Minus One: Parents' Stories of Love & Loss edited by Sean Hanish
and Brooke Warner. $17.95, 978-1-938314-80-3. A collection of
stories and artwork by parents who have suffered child loss that offers insight into this unique and devastating experience.